Looking Upward

Facing and Reaching Beyond Spinal Cord Injury

Ronald C. Schultz, Ph.D.

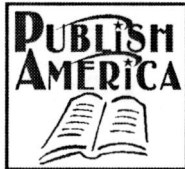

PublishAmerica
Baltimore

First printing

At the specific preference of the author, PublishAmerica allowed this work to remain exactly as the author intended, verbatim, without editorial input.

ISBN: 1-4241-2648-7
PUBLISHED BY PUBLISHAMERICA, LLLP
www.publishamerica.com
Baltimore

Printed in the United States of America

Dedicated to my wife Linda
who helped add meaning to my post-injury life;
to my family
whose support and presence were always there;
to the gift and bond
of true and enduring friendship;
and in remembrance of my brother Ray
with whom I shared so many memorable times
in my pre-injury years.

I. A Night to Remember

Town of Cambria
Niagara County, New York
Monday, December 30, 1968

Tired eyes strain to focus on headlight beams piercing the dark wintry night, as with dull impatience I count off the miles separating me from a few hours of sleep at home. It is late, or early, sometime between midnight and morning. Head foggy; thoughts random; actions mechanical.

Across the seat no sound from younger brother Ray—another mind lost in the twilight of the hour. Wheels turning; distance passing in silence; nothing but destination left.

Boundaries between dreams and nightmares at times easily blend, abandoning safety to peril in an unwarned instant. I drift through this thin wall of opposites and am at once enveloped by a choking mist of impending doom. Startled by a sharp jolt of apprehension, my mind springs to alertness like a trapped prey. Not quick enough—the looming outcome can't be swayed!

Nightmares unfold in a nether land where there is no control, and where what can't happen does. Through an eerie veil I see the guiding path of headlights swing off course as traction suddenly fails on the icy-slick surface of the long, never-ending curve stretching ahead. Brakes and steering wheel useless, it's futile to even try. Real or unreal? I almost can't tell.

Neither gallant deed nor trickery of mind can help us now. The uncontrolled slide continues, assuring this surreal drama of an unwelcome ending. The rear of the automobile whips forcefully around to where the front had been only a moment before, flinging the ill-fated vehicle off the road with vicious momentum. Piled-up ridges of hardened, jagged ice lining the sides of the highway make good on their threatening presence, gashing open the left front tire as it rams into jutting, razor-sharp edges. The car dips sharply and abruptly as the tire blows, and begins to overturn as it leaves the road. Violent thuds and crashes pierce the stillness of the night as the auto, imitating an out-of-control acrobat, tumbles wildly through the darkness. Flung about like rag dolls because there are no seat belts, we are at fate's mercy as the car flips from an upright position onto its side, from its side onto its top, from its top onto its other side, from this position to an upright position once again, and then, still rolling, to a final resting position on its side, driver's side down and passenger's side up.

It all happened so suddenly and is over so quickly, and seems so uncannily unreal, that there is no immediate response from either me or Ray—just empty silence except for the gentle hum of the car's engine, which somehow is still running. Ray is the first to finally speak, chastising me in an "I figured this would happen" tone, most likely because of his rejected offer to drive home, "Well...you'd better turn it off!"

"I can't," is my simple reply, after which Ray reaches and shuts off the ignition switch.

"Are you hurt?" asks Ray.

"You'd better believe it," I answer.

"Are you bleeding?" Ray inquires next.

"No," I reply.

My reactions are matter-of-fact and unemotional. Without knowing exactly what has happened I nonetheless have a clear sense that something is seriously wrong, yet this awareness is in a very passive way. Feelings about what has just occurred are subdued and almost nonchalant. Things are now out of my hands. I have no control over the situation, and the strange thing is I am too detached and physically spent to that much care.

Suddenly Ray becomes concerned, saying excitedly not to worry, that he will get help. Though badly shaken up he seems otherwise uninjured and manages to climb out the window on the front passenger side, which stares blankly into the nighttime sky above. By now I am aware of a growing ache in my neck and ask Ray if he can put something under my head to support it. Removing his jacket, Ray pushes it through the opening where the driver's side door is ajar, positioning it in place as best he can. He then hurries off toward a nearby house to seek help.

What am I doing lying in a flipped over car in some farmer's field in the dead of a winter's night? I should pinch myself to see if this is real. That would be the thing to do, except I can't move. What's going on; what's happened to me? I didn't feel any pain as the auto flipped, just the shock of those heavy, jolting impacts each time the vehicle rudely slammed the ground. Yet something isn't right, because my arms and legs won't move. Are they broken? They feel all twisted and entwined about one another. If I glance downward toward where they are, maybe I can find out what's wrong. No use— it's too dark to see anything. Strangely there is no pain in my limbs, just a weird feeling of nothingness.

Well, I'll just have to deal with this later. Right now I am so tired that I need to go to sleep for a while. Yes, nothing is as important as a deep, long, uninterrupted sleep. As I fall off into the subdued regions of my consciousness, from somewhere far off in the distance the voice of Ray desperately informing someone that there has been an accident and that I need help filters hazily back to where I lay.

After some time, I really don't know how long, I become aware of a bustle of activity at the scene. An ambulance has arrived, but since I can't be removed from the car in its overturned position a tow truck is summoned to upright it. In the meantime a state trooper approaches and fires off a barrage of questions, which I answer mechanically with forced effort.

The tow truck finally arrives and I hear voices discussing a strategy for getting the car back on all four wheels. I just want to get on with it, but soon question the wisdom of the plan when before the auto can assume a fully upright position its controlled descent from its side onto its wheels is lost and the car crashes heavily to the ground. Despite someone standing alongside the auto trying to hold me in position during the maneuver, still the landing shock is jarringly severe. Nonetheless, the vehicle is once again upright and I can now be transferred to the waiting ambulance and be on my way to the hospital.

The ambulance's destination is the small, nearby city of Lockport where I began the evening by picking up Ray. Arriving at the emergency room of the city's sole hospital, the very hospital where I was born, I am met by a sheriff's deputy and questioned once again. I'd rather have these law enforcement people let me be for the immediate time, but I suppose they figured they had a job to do and were going to do it.

I am placed on an examination table and my clothes are removed to allow a full evaluation of my injury. The hospital is small, and nighttime staffing is not like that in larger urban hospitals. There is only one attending physician on duty, and he is already busily working on another emergency. He has to rush back-and-forth between two examination rooms to tend both situations.

X-rays reveal that I have a fractured neck, and orders are given to immediately immobilize the cervical spine by placing a sandbag along each side of my head to keep it from moving. It is unknown how much further damage may have occurred as the result of unrestrained movement from the time of injury up to this point. Unwittingly even I contributed to that upon first being placed on the emergency room's examination table, raising my head to look toward where Ray was being checked over to see if he really was okay. And at the scene of the accident there were no paramedics on hand, so there were no precautionary measures such as securing me to a backboard to prevent movement of the spine. Yet, it was unlikely anyone there had the training to determine that a spinal injury might have occurred. The ambulance attendants meant well and I was grateful for their help, but they were just rural volunteer firemen out there in the middle of the night doing the best they could.

Lacking adequate treatment capability at this hospital for my type of injury, mainly the services of a skilled neurosurgeon, arrangements are made for my immediate transfer by ambulance to a hospital in Buffalo, about 35 miles away. Back on the road; engulfed once more by the night; unwilling hostage to reality. On a desperate mission at a desperate hour, the emergency vehicle feels its way through the night, pulsing with random motion I sense from the edge of awareness during shifts in speed and direction. Suddenly one of the sandbags alongside my head moves and an anonymous voice exclaims with urgency, "Watch those sandbags!"

I feel relief yet at the same time apprehension as the ambulance glides up to the emergency entrance at the hospital in Buffalo. I am whisked directly to the Intensive Care Unit to await the arrival of the neurosurgeon who will handle my case. The clock ticks on—no physician. I become anxious to have the needs of my physical predicament met, to have resolved one way or another the uncertainty surrounding me.

About 7 A.M. the doctor finally appears and immediately reads X-rays of my injured neck. Seeing what needs to be done, he shaves all but the back of my head, injects novocaine on each side of my head towards the back, and then with a hand drill begins to cut two holes in my skull just deep enough to allow a device known as "Crutchfield tongs" to be attached.

A normally unacceptable thing—drilling holes in my skull with a hand drill! Black and Decker? Probably not. Something unthinkable now passively accepted by me because I have no choice. What has happened has happened, and from this point I can do nothing but experience and endure whatever I must.

The Crutchfield tongs resemble a pair of ice tongs clutching the sides of my head, and to them a traction apparatus is attached so that the pull of weights might restore proper alignment of my dislocated spinal vertebrae. When the attachment of tongs and traction is completed, through the blurring fog surrounding me I hear the doctor's simple and blunt pronouncement, "All right, you have a broken neck." He strides over to the nurses' station to write out orders, and then leaves.

9

Family members are now allowed to briefly see me. They are not encouraged. Asking about my condition as the doctor is leaving, my mother is told plainly and abruptly, "If he makes it through the first forty-eight hours we'll talk from there."

Whether or not it should, none of this greatly concerns me. I am sort of half here and half not and in the floating, almost dream-like state I'm in don't very much care what really is going on. All I want is to drift away undisturbed on a distant cloud of sleep. When I awaken this nightmare will be gone, and everything will be the same as before.

II. Can This Be Real?

Secure in a land of dreams where reality has no reign, scenes wisp by that are friendly and responsive to my will. Here all is well, and I may stay forever to celebrate youth, health, happiness and prosperity. Warm feelings; pleasant visions and experiences; confidence and invulnerability. Images begin to focus as suddenly I am reliving Friday night. Alone with someone special in a private domain all our own, there is surrounding silence saturated with sensations and emotions, unspoken testimony to a bond needing no sound except the beating of two hearts to verify its truth. This is my preferred reality and world of choice.

But wait! Another image flushes over this pleasing revisitation as time snaps forward to Sunday evening. Is there no refuge even in my dreams?! The piercing sting of cold winter air chills me to the core, giving evidence to nature's impact on this night following the devastating ice storm that so unmercifully struck our area. Yet youth is adventurous and takes no caution. Ray and I are determined to have our night out, and we are not put off. At ages 19 and 22 we are not mortal or vulnerable beings, but rather bold and undefeatable challengers of fate. We are kings of our destinies and we are in control.

Both eyes snap open as even my subconscious mind refuses to accept the consequences of this folly. Cruelly returned to stark reality, unwillingly my view takes in the sterile hospital surroundings as a silent scream exclaims, "It's true!!"

In whatever transitory realm I had been there was no threat to my mortal existence, regardless of the doctor's somber declaration after attending to me. I would have felt that type of presence and didn't, so that was not in the plan for me. Something else is, though, because here I lay. Once more back among the living I am out of further physical danger, but maybe what I have to deal with now is almost as bad.

The psychological shock is heavy—a transformation in an instant from a normal, healthy, independent person to a state of complete helplessness. This isn't a pleasant fact to have to face. And, I don't even want to think about what lies ahead. I know only that I am trapped by the way things are, and that I have no control whatsoever over what now confronts me.

How can this be? It seems so unreal. No cuts, hardly even any bruises, only a broken neck. Yeah, *ONLY* a broken neck! Ray just banged up a bit, yet myself injured the way I am. Was this freak twist of fate directed solely at me? Whether I deserve it or not that's what must be, because from that same overturned car only Ray walked away unharmed.

My mind keeps pounding away that it doesn't add up, that this shouldn't be. What really happened anyway? Trying to mentally replay the fateful event, I struggle to visualize how, exactly, my injury occurred. I was thrown around as the car flipped, but don't know how much. Since the driver's side door was ajar, I suppose it even was possible that I started to be ejected. Or, maybe Ray fell hard against me, or perhaps my head whipped and my neck struck something in a certain way—I just don't know. Yet everything keeps coming back to the question of why I was injured and Ray not. My original thoughts must be true; regardless of my own portion of blame for what happened, for whatever reason fate singled me out at that moment and dealt with me accordingly. I can't turn time back and change that.

And there, for sure, goes tomorrow night's New Year's Eve celebration—might as well forget about anything as upbeat as that. I should have at least waited until after the much anticipated countdown to do something like landing in the intensive care unit of a hospital. This isn't the way to ring in the last year of a good and memorable decade in my life, or any other year for that matter. I wish all this really was just a bad dream from which I could awaken and have everything be okay again, but in reality I know it isn't so. Aside from this present but totally unwanted personal experience awareness that they can be very incapacitating injuries, I don't know much about broken necks. I remember my sister breaking her wrist years ago when she toppled from the top of a wobbly stepladder and I can still see my brother's arm in that cumbersome, white plaster cast after he tumbled over the edge of a slide at school. Their recoveries didn't take long. But, what about a broken neck? My first real injury, and it has to be a broken neck. Just where do I go from here?

Things have always turned out all right for me before. My mind begins to work as I recall a story about poetic and philosophical folk singer Bob Dylan, who fractured his neck in a motorcycle accident and was in seclusion for about a year afterward. Hopeful and encouraged, I grab hold of this comparison to judge the length of time needed for my own full recovery. I am feeling better already, and am thankful that my health is going to be restored.

But wait—bad news; cruel news; unacceptable news! I soon find that things aren't so simple. True, Dylan broke his neck, but none of his vertebrae dislocated. My injury is a dislocation fracture of the fourth and fifth cervical vertebrae, and my spinal cord has been damaged. That's why I can't move. It is uncertain just how much recovery, if any, I might have or how long it might take.

Well, okay. Maybe I just need time. Yes, time will take care of things and I'll recover. I really don't want to hear or think about anything else. It will happen; I know it will. I'm not going to accept anything else.

III. Welcome to ICU

Being a constant seeker, I was not one for dullness or routine. Life for me always had to have something extra, and if it wasn't there I would go looking for it. I could freely do that before, but it would not happen where I was now. I was a prisoner against my will, in a confining setting without bars except those imposed by my own body. It would truly be a test to see just how well I endured all of this.

Having gotten through the crisis immediately following my injury, the road to recovery, no matter how long and tough it might be, was at least now open. Yet there remained concern about possible complications from breathing difficulties or pneumonia. To minimize this risk, a respiratory therapy program consisting of four 15-minute treatments each day was begun to increase and maintain breathing capacity and administer medication to help guard against lung infection. These sessions were tolerated, not enjoyed, since they always left my throat dry and sometimes I experienced an accelerated heart rate lasting a few minutes after treatment. I soon discovered the accelerated heart rate was likely to occur whenever two treatments were given too closely together, or if too high a medication dosage was administered during a treatment. Fun, fun, fun!

The respiratory therapy treatments worked, and I didn't develop any respiratory problems. Besides the respiratory therapy treatments, I also began receiving bedside physical therapy treatments to help preserve full range of motion in my limbs, prevent the development of muscle contractures, and assist the return of any voluntary muscle control that might occur. First the therapist would passively move my arms and legs through their normal range of motion, and then ask me to concentrate on moving them as he repeated the motions. These sessions I liked, and because of the physical activity they always left me feeling relaxed and thinking that maybe I might start regaining more voluntary movement. As if breaking my neck and being paralyzed weren't enough, it soon became clear that yet another unpleasant experience lay ahead. As soon as swelling in my neck lessened and the dislocated vertebrae were properly realigned, surgery would be required to fuse the vertebrae and relieve pressure on nerves at the injury site.

My own thoughts rejected the necessity of this operation, deeply fearing the unknown aftermaths of the surgery. I had visions of tubes in my nose, neck, and throat and of not being able talk afterward—a total loss of communication and post-surgery inability to have my discomforts, pains, wants and needs known. Maybe I feared getting worse instead of better. How was I to be sure of this frightening procedure—entering that suspended, death-like state of anesthesia and emerging from it in what condition? I dreaded the thoughts of it, yet realistically had to accept that whatever had to be done was going to be done. All I could do was hope for the best when the time for surgery came.

What I most disliked about the Intensive Care Unit (ICU) was its very strict and limited visitation schedule. Time seemed to pass so unbearably slow just lying in bed 24 hours a day doing nothing, and I always looked forward to having someone with whom to visit, whoever it might be.

Usually members of my family came during regular visiting hours, but other persons also stopped by to see me at various times. My doctor or a substitute would pop in to check on me; therapists came to give me treatments; some of the Sisters of the hospital as well as priests stopped to visit; and, also now and then the Lutheran ministers from the communities where I had attended church. Nurses visited and spent time doing things for me, and a couple of students in training at the hospital dropped by to tell me about such things as "prism glasses" and "circular electric beds." Even a patient known as "Joe," who lost one of his legs just below the knee in an auto accident, was allowed into ICU frequently to visit me. Joe was just 25 and married, so his misfortune presented its own problems. Still, he took the time to stop in to see me.

Visiting times, restricted to members of the immediate family, were at two, six and 10 P.M. Each session lasted five minutes—a total of 15 minutes each day—and I could usually forget about the 10 P.M. visitation because it wasn't practical for my family. It was such a long drive for them to and from the hospital, and right in the dead of winter. Driving that distance so late at night in bad weather when physically or mentally fatigued, or both, was a risk.

A further ICU restriction was that only one person was allowed to visit at any given time. There were, of course, some very sick people in ICU, so the restrictions were understandable. I found that quite often the condition of the patient determined the strictness or laxness of visitation rule enforcement.

I was able to have extra visitation time because members of my family were allowed to feed me my lunch and dinner meals, which I was unable to do on my own. This benefited the nurses as well as myself, since it lessened their mealtime patient load by one; it freed someone who was then able to feed or tend another patient who might need some sort of assistance, and there were a lot who did in ICU. I, of course, got to spend that much more time with family members. Regaining the capability of feeding myself, though, was for me going to be one of the first and highest priorities in my rehabilitation, because I wanted to as soon as possible get back at least that much independence.

During those periods when I didn't have visitors, which was most of the time, I could do little more than lie in bed waiting for time to pass. The view of things around me was very restricted, since I had to lie completely flat and could see only the pale-white, pegboard-sectioned ceiling above me and a limited area to each side of my bed. At night I often saw reflected up through the fourth story window next to my bed the flashing red lights of ambulances as they pulled up to the emergency room entrance below. The bright, ruby, pulsating bursts cut sharply through the darkness where I lay, attracting my attention as they bounced off the wall and ceiling near me. These colorful visual displays were a noticeable contrast to the otherwise subdued tones of the night, but each time I wondered who was being brought to the hospital and what their misfortune might be. I always looked forward to visits from an occupational therapy student who often stopped by to see me. She recommended getting a pair of prism glasses and told me how I might do that. I did get the prism glasses, and they helped expand my visual field by enabling me to see in a horizontal direction even though I was lying flat on my back. These fascinating lenses had the same effect as looking through the periscope of a submarine; they bent light at right angles. During my time lying flat in ICU where there was such a restriction on visitation, I got amusement from the glasses since they allowed me to see activities around me from the perspective of an upright person. If I ever got out of here and into a semiprivate room, they might be useful in watching television if I had to continue lying flat for a time.

A persisting and menacing problem was the unrelenting tug of the traction weights attached to my head. The force of these weights constantly pulled me toward the top of the bed where sooner or later my head came into contact with and pressed heavily against the hard metal of the headboard, causing much discomfort. In their thoughtful mercy the nurses would then come and pull me down toward the foot of the bed a ways, and this would be okay for a while until the weights again dragged me up against the head of the bed, once more necessitating the return of the nurses and a repeat of their rescue efforts. But, this was just another of the unwelcome things I had to put up with during the early stages following my injury.

Eventually I was permitted to have a small transistor radio, provided I kept its volume low enough so as not to disturb other patients. I even was allowed to watch Super Bowl III between the New York Jets and Baltimore Colts on a small portable television that was set on the edge of my bed. Although oddsmakers and most everyone else thought differently, three days before the game confident Jets' quarterback Joe Namath stated matter-of-factly, "The Jets will win on Sunday; I guarantee it."

The Jets won. I wished I had the same confidence and certainty regarding the outcome of my physical condition as "Broadway Joe" had about the outcome of football competition. Where were my guarantees?

On the radio I heard such songs as Barry McGuire's "Eve of Destruction," which seemed quite appropriate for me, Sly and the Family Stone's, "Everyday People," and "Games People Play" by Joe South. Yet, I found I could listen to the radio only for a short while before it became annoying. Even though the radio provided at least some entertainment, I wasn't able to get a great degree of enjoyment from it. Considering the total state of things at this time, it seemed somewhat repulsive and unacceptable to think of anything as being enjoyable, and I just was not in a content enough frame of mind to do so. It seemed more appropriate to separate the good from the bad and not mix the two. To me that would be like trying to laugh and cry at the same time.

Now that I was limited physically, a much greater burden was placed on me mentally. I really began to think about things, anything and everything. Particularly, I began to realize that life wasn't always such a sweet bowl of roses—it had a down side as well. And, there's no hiding from that truth; it has to be faced and accepted. If not, it will find you and set you straight. You can't simply wish life into being what you want it to be. Although you have some control, in the end you pretty much have to take it for what it is. You can try to get things to go your way, but there is only so much you can do. The rest is out of your control.

No matter how positive I tried to be, the circumstance I was in left me confused and disorganized and I struggled to get a true grip on reality. I had to acknowledge the despair within me; I had to acknowledge the dismal cloud overhead. The good side of life had suddenly vanished and everything now seemed reversed. Everything was the opposite of what it really should be.

It was unacceptable. I was too young and independent to be facing this type of catastrophe. It was hard to believe, being so self-sufficient one day and totally out of control of my life the next. It shouldn't be this way. Only good things should be happening at this point in my life. I wanted desperately to escape it all—cast it aside and grasp a greater security and reality of my own choosing.

When my life got off to such a promising start, I thought it would stay that way. As the years of challenge and sacrifice of World War II came to an end in August of '45, better times lay ahead for good ol' USA and its people. It was into this forward-looking, optimistic atmosphere that as one of the original post-war "baby boomers" I came into this world on St. Patrick's Day in 1946. I had it made. The luck of the Irish was with me and there would be no stopping me in life. I had arrived at the right time—a time of peace and prosperity when Irish eyes were smiling.

Irish eyes kept smiling right up through my twenty-second year. At this stage of my youth I looked around me and thought what a wonderful place in which to live the world was. It was a time in my life when I was just beginning to realize my true potential and the seemingly endless opportunities that lay before me. I felt as though there was so much ahead of me and so little standing in my way, that I just couldn't imagine anything being contrary to my optimistic view of things. Unable to look beyond my own private realm of being, I was blind to the fact that life is not solely a one-sided experience. As far as I was concerned, the only reality to be acknowledged was that which was right there with and around me. All else to me was merely an illusion—an unreal and inconsequential existence.

Now, though, the luck of the Irish had deserted me. What happened wasn't good luck, so throw the advantage of being born on St. Patrick's Day right out the window. What was left, and what mattered most, was how everything would eventually turn out. Just what would become of it all? To where would it all lead? Was there a way out? Apparently, only time would tell.

I still had one thing to hold on to—hope. At least that was something on which to focus and believe in. It was a very important something that would help motivate me and keep my spirits up.

Hopefully, things sooner or later would get better. Right now they certainly couldn't get much worse.

After being in ICU for nearly a month, I was ready to be transferred to a semiprivate room in another part of the hospital. In one way I was concerned about the move, because in ICU there were always nurses at hand in case I might need something. Once I left ICU, I could expect things to change considerably; I would be much more on my own. Yet on the other hand, once out of ICU visitation rules would become much less restrictive, and I looked very favorably upon that.

I was moved to a spacious, very pleasant room in a newer section of the hospital's fourth floor, to which I took an immediate liking. A radio, television and telephone were all now at my disposal, and I had practically unlimited visitation privileges compared with those in ICU. Plants and flowers were placed by the windows, and cards and posters were put on the walls. All these had been sent or brought to me by friends and relatives, and they helped brighten up the room. This new-found freedom made me a bit more cheerful, and the change of atmosphere seemed to do some good.

IV. To Be or Not to Be

My pre-accident world was one of personal control and invulnerability. Bad things weren't a part of my life, and bleak happenings such as tragedy and death were distant events in the lives of others having no real meaning to me. Now suddenly I found myself in the midst of extreme contradiction; not only had I personally been stunned by a much unwanted life circumstance, but from the inescapable vantage point of my hospital bed the misfortune and even mortal departure of others too crowded in on me from all sides. As a patient in the hospital, I found myself right in the midst of death itself. The Intensive Care Unit in particular, because of its requirements for accepting patients, seemed literally a haven for departing souls. Nighttime regularly set the stage for the morbid drama to begin, whereupon the notorious lead player, in its sinister and shadowy form, invariably stole onto the scene to deal with the chosen cast. An alarmingly large number of patients entering ICU ended up making their grand exit covered by a plain white sheet.

Ambulance calls increased considerably at night, bringing with them the arrival of victim upon victim of various catastrophes. The news of each casualty spread quickly throughout the hospital as word passed among the personnel on duty. I dreaded the nights and always welcomed the reassuring rays of bright, morning sunshine.

I thought the whole mood present in ICU would brighten after my transfer to the semiprivate room I now occupied, and in the beginning it did. My first roommate was in his mid or possibly late twenties, and had been admitted to have knee surgery due to torn cartilage. His hospitalization was only for a short time, too short to get to know him really well, but as a roommate his presence was uplifting. Because of my daily habit of borrowing his portable shaving mirror, he gave it to me when he left, ribbing me that I got more use from it than he ever would.

As the sun rises each morn, saturating the world with renewed hope and optimism, there is freedom of choice to reach out and grasp its golden beams or let them pass by. Sometimes life's light no longer shines brightly, but instead becomes an overwhelming weight too heavy to bear. There are those who fight life's challenges and others who wear down under its burdens and give up. It is a matter of inner feeling and decision that each individual personally embraces, and I was about to come face-to-face with someone who had chosen defeat and resignation.

My second roommate was an older man appearing to be somewhere in his seventies. This man, who I will simply refer to as "Mr. K" in abbreviation of his much longer last name, had been admitted to the hospital for diagnostic tests to pinpoint a suspected bladder or kidney problem. Mr. K was very withdrawn, almost totally unreceptive to the world around him. His wife served as his spokesperson, and he remained mute and expressionless while she did all of his bidding for him. Mr. K seldom talked to anyone, especially his wife, and on only one occasion when an old friend stopped by to see him did he speak and visit openly and possibly even cheerfully. From what I could see, Mr. K seemed to lack any degree of vitality or zest for life.

Mr. K's wife came faithfully each afternoon and evening to visit and be with him, but he almost totally ignored her and said nothing to her unless he absolutely had to. Mrs. K pampered her husband and waited on him with doting care, rambling on continuously all the while, but he remained locked up in his own private, faraway world and paid little attention to her. Mrs. K seemed to have centered her whole world around her husband, obviously to an extreme, and he appeared to merely want to be left alone.

It seemed as if to Mr. K his wife was no less than an ever-present and inescapable catalyst, constantly kindling the fire of discontent burning within him. All I could detect when looking at him was a sense of apathy, despair, frustration, anger and resentment, all turned inward against himself. From what I could tell, Mr. K had given up on life. It appeared he simply wanted life and all of its frustrations to leave him alone. If he couldn't find further purpose in life, then perhaps he felt there was no use even trying anymore. Aside from any physical ailment he might have had, Mr. K's real problem seemed to be his total indifference toward life. Compared to this self-destructive state of mind, Mr. K's physical condition, whatever it might have been, seemed minimal.

Although nothing was found right away, one afternoon while his wife was visiting, the doctor in charge of Mr. K's case came into the room and informed them that the results of Mr. K's tests confirmed the presence of a partial obstruction in the urinary tract that required corrective surgery and then post-surgery bladder catherization for some time. Although Mr. K said not a word, I gathered from the way his eyes suddenly shot open to about twice their normal appearance that he wanted no part of what the doctor had in mind and from this point his withdrawal became even more extreme.

Already in the first days of the very few before his scheduled surgery, Mr. K's steadily increasing boycott on life became more and more evident. He hardly touched his meals; he did not talk to anyone; he maintained and very closely guarded his immobilized state of activity. He did not give one inch in the direction of living. He had made his decision and nothing was going to sway him from his chosen course.

The fateful day started off with the same hospital routine as any other morning. The nurse assigned to our room came in with our breakfast trays, setting Mr. K's on his bedside table and positioning the rollable table in front of him before leaving mine while she took to the other patients assigned to her their trays. The nurse returned and started feeding me my breakfast, all the while urging Mr. K, who completely ignored his tray and disregarded her persistent prodding, to eat something. Mr. K seemed almost catatonic, staring off into space as if in a trance and remaining totally unresponsive to any attempt at communication with him.

After the breakfast trays were taken away, the nurse began our daily A.M. care. She brought Mr. K a basin of water, soap, towel and washcloth, and told him to begin washing himself and that she would be back to give him some assistance after she checked on another patient. Mr. K's unresponsiveness continued as the nurse drew shut the bed enclosures and left.

Since the room divider between our beds was drawn I couldn't see Mr. K, yet he remained strangely silent and inactive. Soon, though, Mr. K suddenly began to breath rapidly and deeply, as if deprived of air and then given access to it again, but this passed rather quickly and I didn't think too much of it. In a short time, however, the same pattern of breathing began once again and once again it stopped after a few seconds.

These were the last breaths I would hear from Mr. K, because when the nurse returned and attempted to get a response from him she discovered that he had, in the words of her later explanation to me, "expired."

Although the nurse said nothing to me at that moment, it didn't take long for me to realize what had happened. I knew the truth but didn't want to believe it, and had to ask and hear it from her plain and simply before I finally accepted it. I couldn't believe someone could actually come to a firm decision to die, and then simply go ahead and do exactly that by focusing a determination that instead could have been used to live.

The tragic thing about this death and what bothered me most, was that it was deliberately self-directed. I was right there all the time watching this man slowly die before my eyes, and there wasn't a thing I or anyone else could have done about it. He simply decided he had had enough of life and would be better off dead. I believe he could have continued living had he really wanted.

Following Mr. K's death, another disturbing event further intensified my confused and uneasy state of mind. Mrs. K, having been informed of her husband's demise, rushed to the hospital and burst into the room in an uncontrollable state of hysteria, unable to cope with what she could not believe had happened. Apparently her life's strength derived mainly from the fulfilled need to provide her husband with an endless and dedicated supply of maternal care and attention, and I believe a part of Mrs. K died along with her husband when the expression of this need was deprived of its long-established outlet.

Although with Mrs. K there was extreme involvement, what happened next appeared to be total indifference. The personnel sent to wrap and take away the body arrived and went about their task in what seemed a very inappropriate and disrespectful manner. One girl in particular laughed uncontrollably all the while as they joked around as if playing some kind of game. Apparently they were unaware of my presence behind the drawn divider, since my bed was on the far side of the room, or if they were aware of my presence perhaps they didn't care anyway.

They acted and carried on as if they were ignorant of the fact, or just downright unconcerned, that someone's life had just ended. Maybe it was defensive behavior for them, a way of desensitizing themselves given the starkness and reality of continually being exposed to this type of assignment. Yet even though it might have been just a routine job for them, it would have affected me much less had they at least shown a little reverence. Their reaction may have been quite different had it been someone close to them. To me the loss of a human life, whoever it might be, was nothing to be made fun of. I couldn't accept this outright display of harshly indifferent behavior, which to me seemed a mockery of the value of life at its worst.

It's a tragedy when persons end their own lives, and hard to imagine the intense internal struggle that brings someone to that point. I had my own psychological battles to wage, and wasn't exempt from feelings of loss and despair after seeing my life change so suddenly and dramatically. Yet, my will to survive and overcome was a counterforce so strong that I wasn't going to give up no matter what.

Personal choice is the deciding factor. You can have a healthy body, but a mind that destroys it. Or, a strong mind can compensate for a physical shortcoming even though this still is not as desirable as having good physical health also. Yet, so much of our lives is influenced by the decisions we make that our inner being really has to be recognized as the true determinant in directing the personal choices of our ongoing life experience.

The Mr. K episode affected me deeply. The entire affair, combined with what I had already experienced up to that point, left me in a disturbed state of mind, and I began to reflect deeply, and somewhat pessimistically, on the very quality and value of life.

Although it may not have occurred under the most favorable of conditions, what I came to realize during the first few weeks in the hospital was something I might not have readily learned under ordinary circumstances. That does not in the least bit mean, though, that I considered my accident to be a valuable learning experience, because I definitely could have done without the injury and what I saw was a bleaker, not brighter, side of reality. I had now been directly exposed to those very forces and events that seem to negate life. My shield of illusion wasn't as impenetrable as it previously appeared to be.

V. Helplessness Is Hell

Unwillingly shackled by the bodily constraints of spinal cord injury, I felt the tremendous psychological impact of being completely dependent on other people. Unable to do anything for myself, I had to totally rely on others for whatever I needed or wanted. I had to be bathed, fed, positioned in bed—I was completely helpless. It was a situation foreign to me, and not one I wanted to accept.

Up to this point, the mainstay of my character had been a hard-earned, self-established ability to be self-sufficient and highly individual and independent. Now, though, I was faced with a complete and extremely disheartening reversal that seriously threatened the very essence of my being. I no longer was capable of guarding my hard-won self-identity, which had so swiftly and unexpectedly vanished like countless grains of sand swept away by a strong desert wind, and I was forced to take a long, deep, inner look at what was now left of me. I was not encouraged by what I saw, and had to fight against falling victim to the dangerously destructive influence of my own self-manufactured despair.

Besides having to deal with the psychological struggles within me, one of my biggest problems was physical discomfort. I had to lie flat on my back with a rolled-up, supporting towel under my neck, turning on either side from time to time in order to prevent skin breakdowns caused by unrelieved pressure on bony areas of my body. Also, because elevation of my head would interfere with proper vertebrae realignment, I was unable to have a pillow. The only comfort for my head was that not so comfortable pair of Crutchfield tongs with its 25 pounds of traction weight relentlessly tugging at me. Thankfully, I learned that the weight was to gradually be reduced, and as this happened it would likely be a great help in lessening the traction discomfort. Another problem was my inability to get rid of excess body heat. As a result of my injury, normal temperature regulation was disrupted. My sweat glands were at least temporarily not functioning, and this left me vulnerable to overheating. Mornings were tolerable, but by late afternoon each day a progressive cycle began whereby within a matter of time I became unbearably warm. Bathing with cold water, applying ice packs— although one time a nurse's aide committed the unforgivable misdeed of using hot water bottles instead—and consuming sherbet and chunks of ice became regular activities in an effort to get rid of built-up body heat. Also, the room temperature was lowered to and kept at a below normal 65 degrees and there was usually a window open even though it was the middle of winter, not a particularly tropic time of year in Buffalo. Many times I wished I was lying outside in a blanket of snow absorbing its cool and refreshing embrace.

It would be several weeks before this overheating problem corrected itself, but as one complication disappeared another popped up. Whereas before I struggled to get rid of body heat, next I swung to the extreme opposite and couldn't retain it, a sort of overcompensation reaction that ironically left me looking for ways to keep warm. It appeared it might be some while before my internal temperature control returned to what might be considered more or less normal. In the meantime, it continued to be a highly hypersensitive system of inappropriate responses.

Getting through the nights during the first few weeks in the hospital also presented a problem. I dreaded the approach of nighttime, for the nights seemed endless and I was able to sleep very little during this time. Unable to relax properly, I was constantly plagued by restlessness, discomfort, excessive warmth, thirst and just plain inability to drift off to sleep. Sleeping pills helped at first but soon lost their effectiveness, resulting in my waking up after only

FACING AND REACHING BEYOND SPINAL CORD INJURY

an hour or two of sleep at most, if I even managed to get to sleep at all. And if I was lucky enough to fall into a good sleep it would be for only a limited time, since my doctor's orders were that my position in bed be shifted every three hours on a 24-hour basis, without exception.

Tension and boredom also plagued me. Boredom was constantly a factor, because I was not one to be restricted in any way. Simply lying around doing nothing was not my idea of the ideal way to spend my time. I readily welcomed each change of position in bed, if only for the sake of the activity itself. Although a high level of comfort was something I seldom experienced, inactivity was no less instrumental in fueling the fire of discontent within me.

Along with boredom was the difficulty of coping with nervous tension. The inability to physically expend energy placed a tremendous mental strain on me. I often became obsessed with the thought that I had to move or change position somehow, and this psychological catalyst was enough to transform tolerable discomfort into unbearable discomfort. I could not see how this would change until I could eventually get out of or at least sit up in bed, whenever that might be.

Although I hoped surgery would not be necessary, it was medically clear from the outset that surgery to fuse the damaged vertebrae in my neck would be required. One Friday approximately four weeks post-injury I was told by my doctor, "We're going to fix you up Wednesday." Surgery was scheduled for 1 P.M.

I was given two pre-operation injections at 11 A.M. on the day of the surgery. These had a very relaxing effect on me and I found it hard to keep from dozing off. Family members stood near my bed talking, for the most part among themselves because I was too drowsy to visit much with them. Eventually a nurse came into the room and said, "They're here for you, Ron."

Two attendants from surgery wheeled me bed and all from my fourth floor room to an elevator that took us up to the fifth floor where surgery was located. The first thing that struck me as we get off the elevator on the fifth floor was the refreshingly cool temperature, apparently a standard condition in surgical areas where temperatures must be kept low enough to minimize bacterial growth. I was wheeled along and then placed outside a large, double-doored operating room at the end of the corridor, where I was left to await the arrival of the surgeon.

It seemed like quite a while before the doctor came along accompanied by some assistants and said, "Let's get him in there." Once inside I was transferred in one smooth, coordinated motion onto an operating table in the center of the room, whereupon my most distinct impression was the size of the huge circular light overhead. Then I become aware of twinges of painful discomfort from the Crutchfield tongs that were still attached to my skull. Someone must have noticed me grimace, because I heard a voice ask how I was doing. I groggily mumbled, "these tongs," and heard the surgeon reply, "We might have to recut those," referring to the niches in my skull into which the tong ends fit.

Next I heard the anesthesiologist say, "a little pin prick here," to which someone couldn't resist the response, apparently referring to the size of the anesthesia needle, "You mean a big pin prick!" Almost instantly I felt an intensely warm sensation flooding rapidly throughout my head. That was the last of which I was conscious until I woke up after the surgery.

According to the surgeon all went well. The damaged cervical disk between the fourth and fifth vertebrae was removed and the two vertebrae were fused at that level. Opposite of what I expected, negative post-surgery effects were minimal and recovery and recuperation were rapid.

I happily discovered that the surgery did eliminate some of the physical problems and discomforts I previously experienced, so apparently there was something to the plan of relieving pressure on nerves at the injury site. Now I began a steady, overall improvement in the way I felt. I also started to sleep much better and was able to endure the nights reasonably well.

Two weeks after surgery the traction apparatus with its remaining five pounds of weight was finally removed. But now that I was free of this, I found myself about to be transferred from my standard hospital bed to an antiquated cast iron piece of equipment known as a "Stryker frame," which had to be dug out of the cobwebbed confines of a storage room somewhere in the basement. This so-called Stryker frame, named after its inventor, obviously hadn't been in use for quite some time and was in a state of complete disassembly. No one knew for sure just how to go about putting it together at first. Assembly took place by trial and error, a small group huddled around the array of parts, each person offering his or her own theory as to what hopefully fit where and what attached to what. After much frustration and a bit of luck, success was finally achieved and I looked with much apprehension at what I was about to be transferred onto.

The Stryker frame was a narrow, stretcher-like apparatus barely wide enough for me to fit on and not much longer than I was tall. It consisted of a main base into which was fitted and locked into place the patient support part of the system. There also was a second identical and interchangeable patient support part. If this second part was fitted over the patient so that the two parts were at the same time connected to the main frame, one below and one above the patient, then when the lock mechanism of the patient support section was released from the frame the patient could be rotated 180 degrees from lying on one's back to a stomach position or vice versa. These two positions were alternated at determined intervals and were the only positions a patient could assume. In my case, position rotation was to take place every three hours.

The distinctive feature of the Stryker frame was its crisscross strips of canvas-like material, interspersed with open spaces, on which the patient lay. This special low surface tension characteristic of the patient support section of the frame, combined with patient rotation at regular intervals, greatly reduced the probability of a patient confined to bed developing skin breakdowns due to unrelieved pressure at bony areas of the body. The Stryker frame was useful in the early stages of cases such as burn or spinal cord injury.

Maybe some patients liked the Stryker frame, but I wasn't one of

31

them. Being turned from one position to the other was a dreadful and disturbing experience, and lying on my stomach on it was sheer agony. Having the top portion of the frame locked down over me in preparation for turning produced an entrapped, claustrophobic feeling. Then, unless the rotation was done in one coordinated, swift movement, which very often did not happen, I would fall awkwardly out of position before the rotation was completed. There probably was a knack to a smooth and uneventful turn of the Stryker frame, but I wasn't the best person to give a good description of it from personal experience.

Lying face down on the Stryker frame was truly an ordeal, and almost never could I remain on my stomach for any great length of time, usually bargaining my way to shorter intervals in this position instead. The reason for my intolerance was mainly that the head support was so uncomfortable. It consisted of two canvas straps, one of which was positioned across my forehead and the other across my chin or thereabouts. Since no one knew too much about the Stryker frame, at first the chin strap was positioned under my chin, causing it to press heavily and uncomfortably against my Adam's apple. Then it was finally decided that the proper place for a chin strap was across the chin, but even this repositioning didn't help much.

The pressure of the head support straps against my flesh, especially the forehead strap, while lying on my stomach became highly irritating and almost intolerable after only a very short time. I had strips of sponge attached to the straps, but this still didn't ease the discomfort. I was always more than ready to be flipped onto my back after enduring a session of lying on my stomach. At least I could relax and be reasonably comfortable lying on my back.

One respiratory therapist I came to like was a young fellow named Jim. Jim was helpful and considerate, and went out of his way to do favors for me. Especially when I was lying on the Stryker frame on my stomach, he would intercede on my behalf and succeeded in getting the nurses to turn me onto my back so I could be given my treatments. Jim could just as simply have left and come back when I was not on my stomach, but he would conspire with me and say "I'll tell them I have to give you your treatment now and they'll turn you onto your back." Then he would leave the room and return with the nurses. Sometimes he even would assist in turning me. For comfort's sake I was grateful to Jim for helping, even though I realized that being turned onto my stomach periodically was for my own good and not intentional torture.

I wish I was able to be as persuasive as Jim with regard to avoiding spending time on my stomach. One day while my father was visiting he offered to go to the snack bar to get a dish of sherbet for me, which at that time I was still consuming frequently in an attempt to keep my body temperature at a cool, comfortable level. Before leaving he told me to make sure the nurses didn't rotate me onto my stomach before he got back with the sherbet. Well the nurses did show up to rotate me, and thinking that a dish of sherbet wasn't a good enough reason to argue against being turned I didn't say anything. This was an example of the type of inconvenience, to say nothing about the discomfort, caused by having to spend time on my stomach on the Stryker frame.

Although my doctor had originally said, "You're going to have to tolerate this Ron," upon becoming aware of my extreme dissatisfaction with the Stryker frame, after only three days on the contraption and constant pleas, he was finally convinced that I had better be taken off the thing before I had a nervous breakdown. The regular hospital bed I was put back into felt like a rock compared to the Stryker frame, but I didn't dare say a word. The bed I had been in before the switch to the Stryker frame at least had a pulsating air mattress, and I wondered why this bed didn't have one also. The answer was that this too was a temporary situation. My doctor had been planning to transfer me to another area hospital because of its physical therapy program, but another reason was its possession of a unique "CircOlectric" bed he hoped to put me in as soon as it became available, and that time was fast approaching.

VI. A New and Different Atmosphere

Although my doctor said I would be transferred to another hospital, I was hardly prepared for the suddenness with which the move took place. I was not told of the transfer until about an hour before two ambulance attendants arrived and entered my room pulling a stretcher. There was barely enough time to gather together my personal belongings and all the other objects accumulated during my 8-week stay at the hospital. There were so many things with which I really didn't know what to do—posters on the wall, flower plants on the windowsill, cards everywhere, and uneaten boxes of chocolate candy that I usually handed out to the nurses—still sitting around. Also, my family had to be notified so they wouldn't show up at the hospital only to find I was no longer there. Taken by surprise, only minimal organization was possible.

The nurses and assistants gathered to say their good-byes and give their best wishes as I was wheeled from my room and down the corridor past the nurses' station to the elevator that would take me to the ground floor a short distance from where the ambulance stood waiting outside. About leaving, similar to my room change I had mixed feelings. I was concerned about having to readjust to the unfamiliar setting of another hospital, yet I was ready for a change—something new and different.

Although quite brisk it was a clear and sunny morning, a most beautiful late February day that seemed to reach out with the message that winter was preparing to give way to the brighter times of spring. After lying flat in bed within the confines of the hospital for two months, with only an occasional glance out the window at not much more than the blue sky above, I was overwhelmed by the

34

extensive visual stimulation that the outside world once again provided. I had an exceptional feeling of well-being as the ambulance hummed smoothly and quietly along the bright, sunshiny streets toward its cross-town destination.

Upon arrival at the other hospital, I was taken by elevator to the south end of the second floor and into a room two doors down from the nurses' station. The room was much smaller and not nearly as new and modern as the one I had been in at the hospital I had just left. There was only one window, and its shade—a dark green roll shade that greatly restricted the entrance of sunlight and reminded me of those my grandmother used to use in her living room to prevent sunlight from fading her upholstered furniture—was lowered all the way. I was instantly overwhelmed by the darkness filling the room, and this bleak atmosphere projected a sharply depressing mood. For a moment reality was transcended as I pictured myself being carried down into the obscure hold of some archaic Nordic castle.

Once inside the room, I was transferred from the stretcher to the CircOlectric bed about which I had heard so much. It was an electrically operated, circular Stryker frame type bed that had just been vacated by a burn patient, thus the sudden short-notice hospital transfer. I immediately took a liking to this unusual and fascinating bed. Not only was it comfortable, but also I felt far more secure than I had in the conventional Stryker frame bed at the other hospital.

The reason for the extreme darkness of the room turned out to be the hypersensitivity of my roommate-to-be to sunlight, or any other type of bright light for that matter. Raising the window shade brought forth from him an immediate and emphatic negative reaction. But when I suggested that the shade should again be lowered his next response was, "The sun will go down." I wondered just what type of roommate with whom I had been teamed, and felt very uncomfortable and as if I'd rather not be in this room. Yet there I was, so for the time being I'd just have to try to make the best of it.

This new roommate, "Sig," was in worse shape than me. He was 24, about a year older than me since in a few days I would be 23, and had been involved in an auto accident six months before mine in

35

which he suffered a dislocation fracture of the same two vertebrae as me, the 4th and 5th cervical. Unfortunately Sig encountered some difficulties that I, by a bit of good fortune and some good care, was able to avoid.

Before coming to this hospital, Sig had been in one in which the care he received showed a degree of negligence. As the result of not having his position in bed shifted at regular intervals, decubitus ulcers—pressure sores of the skin—had developed to the point where plastic surgery repair was needed.

Sig was on a regular Stryker frame and like I had been wasn't fond of being turned in it, especially onto his stomach. At night he often refused to be turned to this position because about his only enjoyment was watching television when nighttime came. He would risk irritating his skin from lying in one position too long, and also provoking the wrath of the head nurse who he would have to face the next morning, and seemed to think nothing of it. Of course that was Sig and his way and everyone sort of understood it, even though they didn't very much like it.

Sig had previously been in the same CircOlectric bed I was now in, but since it turned end-over-end instead of from side-to-side his preference was the conventional Stryker frame. He told me he used to get nauseous and pass out every time an attempt was made to turn him in the CircOlectric bed, and said I was more than welcome to it.

At least the Stryker frame Sig was on was a newer aluminum model, which was a considerable improvement over that ancient, cast-iron relic I had the misfortune of being on at the other hospital. Moreover, it had a whole face mask to support the head instead of just two, thin, torture-producing straps such as I had to endure. The important thing, though, was that Sig could tolerate being turned on the regular Stryker frame, and with his skin condition it was essential that he be turned regularly.

As for Sig and his dilemma, due to the deplorable condition and uncontrollable situation in which he dejectedly viewed himself as being, he had developed an extremely negative and defensive attitude toward everyone and everything with which he came into contact. For sure such a pessimistic and self-defeating outlook was not a healthy or helpful attitude to have when already faced with a severe physical condition, yet the tremendous psychological implications of coping with and adjusting to such a high level, incapacitating spinal cord injury, especially with such serious accompanying complications as skin breakdowns, have to be recognized.

At first there is denial during which there is hope and belief that recovery is just a matter of time, and that the problem will eventually take care of itself. The truth is rejected, because reality itself does not seem real. It is just too unacceptable to be taken as objective fact, and there is a desperate attempt to cling to conditions of the past. But as it is realized that perhaps things aren't going to automatically resolve themselves after all, denial gives way to despair. The mind feels as if it will soon completely shatter, and there is an ensuing fall into the dark abyss of brooding self-doubt and hopelessness.

At this point there are only two ways to go—with it or against it. Yet even if there is an effort to fight back and success is achieved in mustering up the strength of all inner resources, there still is the realization that there is far less control and confidence of outcome than has ever been before. Exactly what is wanted and needed is clearly known, but the self-capacity and power to accomplish that simply doesn't exist. It isn't as easy as just walking away from it all and having everything be the same as before; it's something that's there to stay. The chains that bind are heavy, and all too often it is easier to fall under the weight of that burden than to endure.

With Sig, it was negative acceptance. Things had gone so wrong that he just didn't care anymore. Circumstances were simply beyond his control. No use hoping anymore; no use trying anymore. Why fight something you couldn't beat? Things weren't meant to go right. He was born under a bad sign. The only response left was the negative, hostile, defensive attitude he showed. He owed himself at least that much. Vent the rage! Ease the inner turmoil! Strike back the only way he could! What other way was there to show he still had some control, regardless of how it might otherwise seem? A twisted sense of power and authority; a false sense, but at least some sense, of security and control.

The pressure was really on Sig as he found himself totally helpless and the victim of injustice after injustice. The driver of the car Sig was riding in at the time of his injury not once came to the hospital to see how he was doing. And Sig's wife left him, taking their two children with her. He had no parents or other family members, except for an aunt who seemed to not want to become too involved. Then, of course, there was the deteriorated condition of his skin, caused by the shirking of duty by others, and his inability to do anything about it. Small wonder Sig saw no reason to be optimistic, quite justifiably showing contempt for it all.

He wanted no sympathy, no understanding, just the right to draw back within himself and be left alone. However, he also wanted the right, when the need arose, to project and give expression to his inner feelings of resentment and futility. After all, where could he go from here? Things could only get worse, not better. This is what Sig saw as his reality.

I soon learned the reason for my being placed in the same room as Sig. The strategy was that somehow Sig and I might influence each other for the better. First, it was thought that by seeing someone worse off than myself, I could visualize how much worse things could have been and might consider my situation as being rather fortunate. Second, there was hope that my determination and optimistic outlook might be an incentive for Sig and encourage him to change his attitude.

The plan failed miserably. Sig's liking for the bleak gloominess of the room, combined with his distorted temperament, began to affect me. It just wouldn't, nor even could it, work. Our differences were too extreme. We didn't belong together and I quickly realized I wanted no part of it. I couldn't help Sig, nor could he help me. I was too vulnerable to his negative influence, and had to either escape it or be pulled down with it.

I wanted a bright room with a cheerful and pleasant atmosphere. But most of all, I wanted the freedom to bathe in the optimism that everything would turn out all right for me. I couldn't have all my hope undermined by the destructive forces of Sig or anyone else. I didn't want to become like him and I couldn't help him, because by trying I would only be destroying myself by draining what limited resources I could bring forth in my own fight for survival. I needed more than anything at this time a positive setting within which to wage my struggle for recovery. I would succeed no other way.

When it became clear that things weren't going to work out to anyone's advantage, I was moved to a spacious, bright and pleasant room at the opposite end of the corridor. Moreover, I found myself with an equally pleasant middle-aged man, a Mr. Boyle, as my new roommate and once again I was in good spirits.

Surprisingly, I was not rotated onto my stomach in the CircOlectric bed and that suited me just fine. My resting positions were on my back and on either side, with other position options being both sitting and standing. And, best of all, it was now time to begin getting out of bed and into a wheelchair.

One of the advantages of the CircOlectric bed was that it could be adjusted to allow the person in it to either sit up or even stand upright if it was desired. After only a day or so in the CircOlectric bed, I was given the okay to start experimenting with various sitting, then standing, positions to see what I could tolerate. If this went well, the next step would be getting out of bed and into a wheelchair. Happy to say, aside from a few brief episodes of becoming a bit lightheaded, I adjusted well to these preparatory exercises and soon was ready for a try at the wheelchair.

Transferring from bed to wheelchair involved a rather ingenious yet simple technique whereby the bed itself assumed the brunt of the work. The transfer merely involved placing a canvas sling under me, hooking it to an overhead bar attached to the bed frame, then placing the bed in a sitting position and rotating it electronically until I descended and was swiveled gently into the awaiting wheelchair at the foot of the bed. It was similar to descending from near the top of a Ferris wheel to the ground below. Actually, the structure of the CircOlectric bed did somewhat resemble a miniature Ferris wheel.

Transferring from wheelchair back into bed simply involved reversing the procedure, since the bed could be revolved in a reverse as well as forward direction.

My first day of wheelchair sitting was limited to 15 minutes, and then as each day went by this was increased as my tolerance allowed so that I could remain up for increasingly longer lengths of time. In the beginning, of course, there was a limit to what I could endure physically. Until I regained more stamina, if I stayed up too long at one time I became fatigued. The two inactive months spent in bed meant that I now needed to go through a period of physical readjustment to being up again.

As for my new roommate, Mr. Boyle, he was friendly and helpful, even going so far as to urge me to wake him up in the night if I needed anything from the nurses. In the middle of one night I began to experience some discomfort and Mr. Boyle became aware of it. That was when he told me to please let him know whenever I needed anything, no matter when it was, and insisted I do that even to point of becoming a bit upset about me failing to do so.

Mr. Boyle also had suffered a neck fracture as the result of tripping and falling headlong down the cellar stairs of his home, ramming his head into a doorjamb at the bottom of the stairs, but fortunately the break involved only a compression hairline fracture so the vertebrae did not dislocate and cause damage to his spinal cord. Because of the injury it was necessary for Mr. Boyle to wear a strap-on head collar traction device, though he often took off the collar for relief until someone with authority came into the room and urged him to put it back on.

Mr. Boyle didn't like the traction apparatus at all, claiming that a couple of loose teeth even resulted from the ordeal. But after a few very trying weeks in traction, with a follow-up period of wearing a cervical support collar, he was able to leave the hospital in fairly good health once again—a happy ending for a well-deserving fellow.

My own situation was that I was in a general hospital where patients typically had acute conditions requiring relatively short stays. My condition, though, wasn't something dealt with in such a short time, so my hospitalization continued while a parade of roommates came and went. After Mr. Boyle, my next roommate was a young amateur hockey player from the Buffalo suburb of Tonawanda named Tom. Tom had a back problem requiring hospitalization and testing. He was easygoing and likeable, and it didn't take long for us to become good friends.

Tom was reading *Playboy* magazine one day and wanted to show me some of the pictures. I didn't want to do that, but couldn't come right out and tell Tom to get them away from me. The pictures made me uncomfortable; I couldn't relate to them. The women had perfect bodies meant for perfect men, and I wasn't one of them. What I was looking at was alien to me, and only reminded me of the very valuable thing I had lost—my youthful health. I wanted to say to Tom, "This isn't part of the world I now have!" but could only remain silent until he finished flipping through the pages.

Tom had a very attractive wife who came to visit each day. He didn't need *Playboy* magazine, because he could spend as much time as he wanted looking at her. I envied Tom. He would be going home soon, where he'd be able to resume a normal man-woman relationship with his beautiful wife. Would I ever have that? My reality was much different, born from the cruel fate of having broken my neck.

After Tom's discharge from the hospital, I was again moved to another room a bit closer to the nurses' station where I found myself with a new roommate, Ed. Like Tom, Ed also had a wife and had his own approach regarding her. Ed fell off a roof, breaking his pelvis, and was now in a full body cast. When Ed's wife showed up to visit him, he kidded her about how he was going to make up for lost time once he got back home with her. She just laughed and said she'd like to see how he was going to do that, since although the cast was going to be cut down some before Ed left the hospital, he still would be going home with a substantial body cast. Ed's simple reply was, "I'll find a way."

I don't know about his wife after he went home, but while he was in the hospital Ed did find a way to have his beer. He had his doctor write a prescription for it and leave it with the nurses so he could have beer in the evenings. Ed's beer was kept in a refrigerator in the room next to the nurses' station, and when he asked for some it was brought to him. Ed was someone who, if he wanted something, could figure out a way to get it. I for sure would have spent a lot of time taking lessons from him if I thought pure persistence and determination could reverse the physical effects of my spinal cord injury, but I wasn't convinced I could simply will myself a fully restored spinal cord no matter how badly I might want that.

Aside from Sig, only one other patient was the wrong person to have as a roommate. This was a senile, elderly man who had to be tied down in his bed to keep him from getting up and wandering away. The minute the nurses brought him into the room I knew he shouldn't be there. He was tied down, but freed himself shortly after and went over to my dresser where he started to take out my clothes. I activated the signal switch to the nurses' station and they came to see what was going on. I was insistent in telling the head nurse that either me or the other person was going to be leaving the room; I didn't care who. The man was transferred elsewhere, and I wasn't paired with a questionable roommate a third time.

I didn't have any problem with a young hypochondriac as a roommate. At least he was of rational mind, and all I had to do was have a sympathetic ear to gain his favor. I also got along well with a middle-aged Jewish man who had been in one of the Nazi concentration camps during World War II. However, one evening one of the orderlies, Pete who was studying for the ministry, decided to give me a late night shave with an electric razor and we were talking and laughing a bit besides. Since it was after bedtime, suddenly from the other side of the room came a loud and emphatic, "Shhh!!" Apparently, we were being told to settle down and call it a night. I guess I couldn't very well complain about roommates if I had a few faults of my own.

Pete was a good guy, though. On his nights off he would sometimes do things like stopping by with a pizza. He was a people-oriented person, so vocations such as either the health care field or the ministry were well suited for him.

Bill was another orderly who like Pete worked the 3 to 11 P.M. shift. Bill took me on tours of different parts of the hospital, from the basement right up to the roof itself. At the very top of the hospital was a sewing room that provided a sunny workplace for the Sisters during the wintertime. Access to the hospital's roof was provided by a door in the sewing room. Through it Bill took me out onto the roof where we could look out upon the outside city area surrounding the hospital. It was a much more free and expanded perspective than the more restricted one offered from inside the hospital only. Gazing off wistfully into a dreamy and endless vista of blue, the temptation was to soar away unfettered into the boundless stretch of sky, and I'd have done it if I had wings.

The nurse in charge on the 11 P.M. to 7 A.M. shift, Bertha, was an older German woman with a matching strong German accent. Being somewhat eccentric in her actions and spouting forth incoherent babble, she would suddenly appear in the room probing the dark with penetrating streams of flashlight rays instead of switching on the overhead or bedside lights. Bertha was energetic and efficient in her work, and quite humorous in kidding around with me. I wondered how anyone could be so vigorous and amusing in the dead of night, and found the answer in the old work ethic and dedication she showed.

Eccentricity of a very pleasant sort existed on the day shift also. Marsha was an exceptionally good-looking, young blond nurse somewhat offbeat in manner but to me most likable nonetheless. What others might have seen as her peculiarities seemed to set her apart and made her strangely appealing in a unique and unexplainable way. Because of Marsha's attractiveness, Bill, the orderly on the 3 to 11 shift, took notice of her. Upon reporting to work one day, with an almost irresistible interest he asked me about Marsha, while at the same time showing an obvious apprehension about her differentness.

I had no problem accepting and relating to Marsha, and because of that she seemed comfortable when interacting with me. Marsha liked to go to the horse races at Buffalo Raceway and even offered to place a bet for me one night, which of course I didn't win. I wasn't at all familiar with the horses and the one I picked naturally did an excellent impression of a tortoise. The raceway would have loved having me as regular bettor. Marsha couldn't be beaten in her wagering as easily, because she was much sharper in her knowledge of the horses.

Elaine was another young and good-looking nurse on the day shift, but much more conventional and down-to-earth than Marsha. I was on a high protein and calcium diet, and was encouraged to consume between main meals things like hamburgers, liquid gelatin and ice cream. Elaine was assigned the duty of taking me down to the snack bar in the basement of the hospital afternoons where I usually would have an ice cream sundae. I guess there were worse ways to while away time in the afternoon than sharing ice cream and company with someone like Elaine.

Overall, 3 to 11 P.M. was the best shift. The official activities and business of the day were largely over, and most of the authority figures were soon gone until morning. Late afternoon and the evening were times to start relaxing and just biding time until the start of the next day. Interaction with the staff on this shift was usually enjoyable and informal. There was one person in particular who stood out above all others and to whom I took a special liking. This was a nurse's aide named Sue, and she would play an important role in the early phases of my post-injury life.

VII. Getting Into the Swing of Things

Now that I was able to be out of bed each day I was anxious to begin going down to the basement floor where the physical and occupational therapy departments were located, for a rigorous schedule of therapy activities. Up to this point the physical and occupational therapists had been coming to my room where I received treatment in bed, or in the wheelchair if I happened to be up. But these sessions could achieve only limited results, and I needed to go directly to the therapy departments to receive maximum treatment benefits.

I finally got the okay to start going to the therapy departments for a complete program of daily treatments. It was good just to get off the second floor and be somewhere else for a change.

My daily physical therapy routine consisted of various mat exercises, both on my own and with the assistance of a therapist. These included sit-ups, sitting balance, rolling practice, and passive and resistive motion exercises. Also, using different pulley setups I was able to work with weights to develop greater strength in those muscles that still functioned.

Unlike physical therapy, which involved working with the whole body, occupational therapy (OT) focused solely on the upper extremities. In OT I again worked with weights, as well as other resistive devices, to strengthen functional upper extremity muscles. I also practiced personal grooming and other activities.

There soon was a problem with my morning OT session. I began missing it because I was not out of bed and ready when the OT assistant came to pick me up. My OT therapist voiced her concern to the floor staff. A compromise was worked out whereby my morning

OT session was scheduled a half hour later, provided that whoever was assigned to assist me each morning would make a good effort to see that I was ready when it came time to go to OT. Surprisingly, I got return of an extensor muscle in each wrist approximately three months post-injury. This was first detected by my OT therapist, and since she did not expect it because of the level of my injury she expressed amazement saying, "Hey, that's not supposed to happen!"

My doctor, though, did hope for some return as the result of the surgery he performed, and he would periodically check on me to see if anything had improved. He would come into my room and say, "Let's see what you can do as far as movement is concerned; let's see you move your toes."

One day while my brother Ray was visiting, I told him I thought I could move my fingers and asked him to watch for movement while I tried. When I tried earlier while alone it felt as though my fingers had moved, but now Ray said he couldn't see any movement. Just about this time my doctor walked in with another physician at his side and asked if I had any new movement. I told him I thought I could move my fingers, to which he replied, "Okay, let's see what you call movement." Well, I tried and again nothing happened. The doctor didn't have much of a reply to this, and I felt a bit foolish after he left the room. It was just my mind playing tricks on me.

On another occasion the doctor asked me to put my arms straight up in the air while I was lying flat on my back in bed. This I did to his surprise, quite successfully, but it was assisted by triceps muscle spasticity that kicked in at that moment. At this time I really didn't have predictable voluntary control of my triceps muscles, except that I could often trigger muscle spasm activity to assist triceps function. Since I had at least successfully done what the doctor asked, I felt good about it and let it go at that. To me an assisted accomplishment was better than no accomplishment at all.

Continuing his periodic inquiry, after being away from the hospital for a few days on an out-of-town trip, I overheard the doctor stop the head nurse in the corridor just outside my room before coming in to see me and ask, "Has he gotten any return?"

My physician was noticeably reserved in his bedside manner and not exceedingly outgoing in communicating with patients, but as for his medical knowledge and skill he was exceptionally good and that's what mattered most to me. He didn't openly reveal a lot to me regarding my condition. One day I asked to what extent was my spinal cord damaged and he replied, "There's no way to look inside a spinal cord to see how badly it's damaged," an accurate assessment for the year 1969.

I wanted to learn more about the effects of traumatic injury on the spinal cord, so I had someone purchase for me at the University of Buffalo bookstore a medical textbook on neuropathology. The neuropathology book was lying on my bedside stand one day when the doctor came into the room to check on me. The book immediately caught his eye and he perked right up and said, "Neuropathology— what are you interested in?"

I replied, "Nothing in particular; I'm just trying to find out a few things."

The doctor then went back to his usual reserved self, but I really captured his interest for a moment. To me it indicated he was very much into his medical specialty.

I was both glad and fortunate that the physician I had was a skilled and knowledgeable surgeon. The surgical procedure he used was a more complicated but superior procedure using an approach through the front rather than the back of the neck, where there are so many muscles and nerves. He did a great job, and having a doctor like him was a big advantage for me. I suppose an outgoing personality and open bedside manner are important enough in their own right, but when it comes to my health my first concern is having the most skillful physician available.

As for my continuing progress in occupational therapy, after initial upper limb strengthening I next learned, with the aid of cuffs, braces and splints at first, to type and feed myself. But, things suddenly took a less favorable turn when differences developed between the administration and my OT therapist Judy regarding whether I should remain at this hospital or transfer to a specialized rehabilitation center. This resulted in Judy leaving the hospital and the OT department shutting down altogether. It wasn't a very large department to begin with—only one licensed part-time therapist, Judy, and a couple of assistants.

I don't know how long the OT department remained non-operational, perhaps just until a replacement for Judy could be found, because I would be the next to go. The OT department shutting down and Judy leaving became a critical event for me in evaluating my status as a patient at this hospital.

It was Judy who was mainly responsible for my transfer to a large, specialized rehabilitation center near New York City. Even though her efforts and straightforward advice on my behalf were in conflict with the head administrator of the rehabilitation wing, nevertheless Judy persisted in helping me realize the goal of going to a major rehabilitation center where I could receive the most benefit. For this I was and always will be grateful to her, because it would turn out to be an invaluable experience for me and was what I really needed at this time. Thanks Judy, wherever you are!

VIII. Face Reality

This above all: to thine ownself be true,
and it must follow, as the night the day,
thou canst not then be false to any man.

From Polonius's farewell to Laertes
in Shakespeare's *Hamlet*

It wasn't long before I became disillusioned with the stance taken by the administration of the hospital's rehabilitation wing. There was such a constant barrage of "Face reality, accept reality," that those words continued to faintly ring in my ears at nighttime. Everything was direct, uncompromising fact taken straight from medical textbooks. I had a C4-C5 spinal cord injury and so "this," and "this," and "this" automatically had to be. I would need "this," I would need "that." No "mights" at all, just all "woulds."

There was too much assumption. There was an attempt to lay it all before me in unchangeable terms, while I still believed in the changeable. I was being forced too soon to accept something I was not yet ready or willing to accept. To me it seemed such a short time since the accident, considering the lengthy period of rehabilitation involved in injuries such as mine. I wanted to go forward with the most positive and optimistic attitude possible—keeping in good spirits; devoting myself to improvement; hoping for the best.

I saw nothing wrong in setting goals higher than I might be capable of achieving. There would be plenty of time to resign myself to the worst later if I had to, but right now I wanted to have a forward outlook and didn't want, nor was I about to, let anything interfere

49

RONALD C. SCHULTZ, PH.D.

with this way of thinking. What was wrong with starting off with hope, effort and determination? If things didn't turn out the way I wanted and expected, then I'd adjust accordingly after honestly evaluating just what had and had not been accomplished. No endeavor ever becomes successful by immediately surrendering to the hopelessness of the situation.

I was told too soon, from my point of view, that the physical limitations of my condition necessitated getting and using an electric wheelchair, a mechanical patient lift (Hoyer lift), and a pair of carbon dioxide, gas-operated hand splints. Supposedly, the electric wheelchair would be required because I would need every bit of energy and couldn't afford to waste it on the physical exertion of pushing a conventional wheelchair by hand. The Hoyer lift would be needed because of similar thinking that my arms would never be strong enough for unassisted transfers to and from a wheelchair. The gas-operated hand splints would supposedly be needed to make it possible to write and perform other manual tasks. All this, and yet it was just 16 weeks since the time of my injury.

I didn't agree. I couldn't allow myself to become dependent on these devices without first giving myself the chance to try to develop the capability of functioning without them. It was just that simple to me, and I was unwilling to have it any other way.

The suggested adaptive equipment was recommended to my insurance company, and the company was ready to provide the devices upon my approval. After continually being approached by the rehabilitation administration about the need for the equipment, I finally gave in and agreed to the acquisition of the electric wheelchair and Hoyer lift, to be provided after I left the hospital. Still, I was determined to avoid relying on them unless the limitations of my physical capabilities made it absolutely necessary. Among my goals were to use a manual wheelchair and work out a way to do wheelchair transfers without the aid of a device such as a Hoyer lift. Also, I wanted to try to do manual tasks without the help of any type of hand splints or braces.

I don't mean to be too chastising, because the hospital

administration had its own ideas on how to rehabilitate spinal cord injured persons and certainly had a right to pursue those ideas if they were thought to be correct. Yet I had a right too, a right to do what I thought was best for me and merely wish to emphasize that a person should never passively settle for less than he or she actually can have.

There comes a time when everyone has to accept the reality of his or her own situation if that is inescapable, but only when it is indeed true reality and not a false representation. Sometimes the appearance of reality can be mistaken for the real thing.

People have to be their own judges at times, searching within themselves to find answers to difficult questions, and have to emerge with at least some awareness of their true wants and needs, as well as their potential for achieving them. This is all anyone can do, and this was all I could do at this time. I owed myself that kind of inner evaluation. I owed myself the effort to try to accomplish all I was capable of achieving. To be true to myself, I couldn't simply give in to the situation and become unquestioningly accepting of premature conclusions.

Time would be the real judge of who was correct. Right now, though, I was not ready for any predetermined, black-and-white declarations of, "This is the way it is, and this is the way it will be for the rest of your life." I'd face and accept reality, yet in my own time and way. But, it wasn't something that could just be handed to me and taken as fact without question. In the end, I had to work it through on my own. It was the only way I could, and would, do it.

51

IX. Off to West Haverstraw

With growing seriousness I had been thinking about transferring to a major rehabilitation center specializing in the treatment of my type of injury ever since Judy, the now departed occupational therapist, first introduced me to the idea. It was obvious that the hospital I was now in, or any other general hospital for that matter, was not the proper or most beneficial place for someone in my condition.

Basically, a general hospital is exactly what the term implies— general in the sense that it is designed for general treatment and does not extensively focus on an intensified, comprehensive program in just one particular area of care. I seemed out of place and felt I rightly belonged in a specialized rehabilitation center designed to deal totally and exclusively with my type of medical situation. It was now time to move on to that sort of setting.

My intentions were no secret, but as it became more and more apparent that I might actually follow through with the transfer, I began to experience resistance against it. Because of the rapid progress I was making, as well as my strong and focused determination, the administration was convinced I had good rehabilitation potential. Besides Sig, I was the only other spinal cord injury patient on the rehabilitation wing. Sig wasn't reaching many rehabilitation goals, and in the absence of family and friendship support the future did not look well for him.

It was hoped I would accomplish much and eventually leave the hospital successfully rehabilitated. The rehabilitation program meant a lot to those in charge, and there were at this time plans for a new rehabilitation wing to be added onto the hospital in the near future. I certainly wished this project success, but felt that at the present time there was limited benefit in my staying and was not willing to sacrifice the full potential of my forward progress in doing so. I needed to get away. I needed to go on to something else, something more advanced. I was ready for it.

It was continually impressed upon me that just as much could be done for me where I was as at any rehabilitation hospital, but I didn't see how that could possibly be. The occupational therapy department was no longer in operation, and the physical therapy department was limited in both personnel and facilities. In talking with one of my physical therapists, he agreed more could be done for me within the specialized setting of the rehabilitation center where I wanted to transfer, then added, "…but don't let anyone know I told you that."

Apparently, the physical therapist had no desire for a repeat of the occupational therapist episode. With her uncompromising honesty Judy initiated the rehabilitation center issue and did not back away from her position, even though it placed her job in jeopardy. I could only respect and admire someone like her, because she had my best interests in mind and didn't sacrifice her principles in the face of greater authority.

Besides the opinion conveyed by administration that there would be no difference in therapeutic treatment at a rehabilitation center, I was cautioned against various pitfalls and disadvantages that went along with the setup and operation of a large-scale rehabilitation facility.

I was told that a while back there was another spinal cord injured patient who had left to go to one of the rehabilitation centers I was considering and not liked it at all. It was said that he returned to the hospital in Buffalo and was eventually discharged successfully rehabilitated. A meeting was set up between this individual and myself so that he might share some of his experiences with me, and also so that I could see his van and electric wheelchair and discuss with him the setup that enabled him to function most efficiently in his daily living.

The meeting did more harm than good. I was not ready for what

I saw, and found myself not able to identify at all with this person. He was an image of which I didn't want any part. I was seeking a self-image as close to physical normalcy as I could get, not a scenario of what was now being presented to me—a scenario in which no further physical improvement would occur. I just didn't believe that in the long run I would end up in the same category as this. I still was strongly rejecting all images that were being handed to me, and wanted desperately to leave all of that behind.

More than ever I was now convinced that I had outgrown the hospital where I now was, and rightfully belong in a specialized rehabilitation center. I needed a more supportive and self-identifying environment in which to be and improve.

As my occupational therapist Judy first suggested, I wrote to New York State Rehabilitation Hospital at West Haverstraw for information. Additionally, I contacted the Institute of Rehabilitation Medicine (IRM) at New York University Medical Center, because I had talked to an occupational therapy student who had interned there and was now proudly taking a position as an OT therapist at another hospital in Buffalo.

Upon telling my doctor that I wanted to transfer to a rehabilitation center, he replied that if that was what I wanted to do he would help in any way he could. He said New York State Rehabilitation Hospital at West Haverstraw, the rehab facility toward which I was leaning, was probably as good a place to go as any.

I did choose West Haverstraw, located along the Hudson River north of New York City, because it was closer and not in a central urban setting such as IRM in Manhattan. This would make travel by anyone from my home area of Western New York State easier. Luckily I had excellent private insurance coverage that would pay fully for my stay at West Haverstraw, as well as my stays at both hospitals in Buffalo, because when I started working for Carborundum Company in Niagara Falls in the fall of '68 I opted for both major medical and disability coverage.

After much conferring, corresponding and coordinating, everything was finally set for my transfer to West Haverstraw. In one sense I would miss those who worked with and befriended me and to whom I had become unavoidably attached, but I was ready and anxious to move on once again to something new and different, hopefully with more promising opportunities. I had always been a strong advocate of the adage, "All nature abhors a vacuum," and always resisted stagnation when change and opportunity were the alternative.

The day of departure was Monday, July 7, just after the Fourth of July weekend during which I was allowed to spend a limited period of time—daytime, not overnight—at home. Travel was by airplane out of Buffalo airport.

It was an exceptionally clear, warm and sunny morning when the American Airlines flight lifted off from Buffalo airport, but 55 minutes later when the plane touched down at Newark it was damp and overcast with a fine, misty rain steadily falling. I hoped this was not a symbolic foreboding of things to follow in my new venture.

Soon after the other passengers get off, an older dark blue vehicle vaguely resembling an ambulance crept to a stop near the foot of the stairs leading up into the plane and stood motionless amidst the damp, persistent drizzle. It was my transportation to the hospital.

The rain continued all the way to West Haverstraw, a trip of about two hours, more than twice as long as it took to fly from Buffalo to Newark. Arriving at the hospital, the rain kept falling in the same steady, fine mist. The roadway leading from the main entrance up to the summit upon which the hospital sat was exceedingly steep, and the out-of-date ambulance labored to ascend it. We continued along a one-way road encircling the hospital and came to a stop barely a stone's throw from the point where we first came in.

I must have been quite a sight as I entered the building on the ambulance stretcher, because due to the rain I was covered head-to-foot with a dark-green hospital blanket and most likely more closely resembled a cadaver than a living being. We entered a ward, and I was taken to my assigned space of residence.

On this first night at the hospital, a well-known research

neurologist came to see me. He interviewed me and gave me a neurological examination. I was ready to begin the slow, gradual process of becoming fully adjusted to this new environment, and working toward whatever degree of functional improvement I could achieve.

X. The Rehab Hospital

The small community of West Haverstraw lay quietly nestled on the west bank of the Hudson River about 50 miles north of New York City. Like a posted sentry, perched atop its elevated land mass overlooking the river the rehabilitation hospital peered down on the picturesque basin below and basked luxuriously in the cool summer breezes that blew gently across the Hudson Valley. These breezes were especially refreshing at nighttime when the sultry, stagnant heat was hardest to endure. The hospital wards were not air-conditioned and the evening winds supplied their own natural cooling, providing comfort and protecting against long, sleepless nights.

The two-story hospital had open wards instead of individual rooms for patients. I was put in Ward A&B, the men's spinal cord injury ward. It had two identical wings separated by a nurses' station and hallway leading out to the main hospital corridor.

For my living space I was assigned a "cubicle" on the east side of the ward, and from the dayroom at the ward's far end one could look out toward the Hudson River and also see traffic coming up onto the hospital grounds from winding Route 9W below running north and south alongside the river.

The wings of Ward A&B were identical in design and setup, having twelve glass-partitioned cubicles, six to a side with a central aisle running down the middle. The cubicles were open-faced to the aisle but had curtains on side and front tracks that could be drawn for privacy. Each cubicle measured about eight by ten feet. Basic furnishings consisted of an electric bed, a tall metal locker for clothing and other personal belongings, a small three-drawer dresser

57

that also served as a nightstand, and a little brown metal folding table that could be used at mealtime or for reading and writing while in bed. I added a small washstand to my cubicle, which was the third cubicle down from the nurses' station on the south side of B wing.

Outside, attached to and running the length of A&B, was a railed cement patio accessible from a door in the dayroom at each end of the ward, as well as from the front door leading outside onto it from the nurses' station. Also, the patio could be accessed through window-doors in some of the cubicles bordering it on the south side of the ward. Some of these doors no longer opened easily because weathering had caused them to warp, or else they had in another way become misaligned, but those that did open gave a direct and easy access to the outside right from the ward itself.

The dayrooms at the end of each wing were large, serving the dual purpose of recreation area and dining facility. There was a black-and-white television in each that if patiently adjusted provided tolerable viewing, and vacant stretchers, wheelchairs and other equipment were usually scattered idly about. Most of the remaining space was taken up by tables and lounge chairs.

Bath, shower, toilet and sink facilities were located in two spacious rooms that ran off the corridor dividing the ward's two wings. Also situated just off this corridor were a medical and drug supply room, utility room, small kitchen, two isolated rooms that could be used for patients under special circumstances or other reasons, an office for the doctors in charge of the ward, and a couple of storage rooms plus a linen closet. There was a pay telephone near the end of the corridor, to which the patients and ward personnel had access.

Although Ward A&B was my home base, there was much more beyond it. The defining feature of the hospital was its ability to integrate the needs of the different wards within it and render effective rehabilitative services accordingly. Patients leaving their wards in various locations in the hospital needed easy access to all services throughout the building, and the setup of the rehab center provided this convenience quite well.

The physical layout of the hospital was unique. Its main rectangular shape was like a big circle, so a person could begin traveling at any point in the main corridor and after going its full distance end up right back at the starting point. This gave easy access to each hospital service and facility, since they all were located just off this main corridor. And if you had to travel a ways to your destination, instead of turning around and going all the way back you could simply continue on around what was left of the circle.

Besides Ward A&B, there were four other wards in use. Ward C&D, the women's spinal cord injury ward, was located on the second floor directly above A&B. Comparing the two wards clearly showed the hazard of being male. Spinal cord injury occurs much less frequently in females because of their lower risk style of living, so the number of spinal cord injured patients on Ward C&D was small, with women having other conditions filling the rest of the ward.

Women's ward E&F and men's ward G&H were at the opposite, west end of the hospital. Similar in setup to the spinal cord injury wards, these wards housed a conglomerate of patients having conditions such as stroke, amputation, brain injury, multiple sclerosis and cerebral palsy.

The final active ward, Ward K, was a children's ward with very young and impressionable children needing special care and attention. It was a very spacious, single-room unit opening directly onto the main hospital corridor. Located at the northeast corner of the hospital away from the other wards, Ward K thrived happily alone by itself in its unique isolation. There was a large, vacant double ward on the floor above Ward K, in use in previous time but unoccupied now.

Although A&B and C&D were primarily spinal cord injury wards, often patients were mixed for reasons of facility or compatibility. For instance, there were three amputees and a person with nonfunctional hips on Ward A&B. There also was someone with a spinal cord tumor on the ward. Age grouping was a big factor, almost all of the guys on our ward being fairly young.

Probably the most important unit of the hospital was the physical therapy department. It was a very large and extensive complex taking up an entire wing at the northwest corner of the hospital. Also quite large and well-equipped was the occupational therapy department, although nothing near what physical therapy was. Occupational therapy was located just off the main corridor in the southwest section of the hospital.

Starting at the point in the main corridor just outside Ward A&B and completely circling the hospital, other services and facilities were: Gift shop; administrative offices and admissions; pharmacy; hospital laboratory; urology; dentist; surgery and medical supplies; X-ray; outpatient clinic; hospital records; recreation department; CP (cerebral palsy) department; music room; library; auditorium-gymnasium; education and counseling (psychology and social services) departments; occupational therapy offices; and, hospital personnel dining hall. One floor below the central part of the hospital was a vocational training department, apparatus department, sewing department, kitchen and small dining area, and storage.

Physical plant and laundry were in a separate building away from the main hospital structure. Residence for student nurses and therapists, as well as for other hospital personnel, also was in separate buildings on the hospital grounds.

Interior to the main rectangular hospital structure was an open outdoor plaza of shrubs, trees, grass and walkways. Near the center of this outdoor area was a fountain that no longer worked, and off to one side was a playground that the kids from Ward K could use.

The outdoor plaza was accessible by several doorways along the main hospital corridor, and there even was a roadway running crossways through the corridor and out into the inner square that grounds maintenance crews used. Using the many available doors spaced out along the corridor, I liked the direct unrestricted access to the inner square where, whenever I wanted, I could go with visitors, staff, or other patients to talk and absorb warm, golden rays of sunshine during the day and stimulating fresh air at night.

At the two roadway through areas in the corridor were large

overhead electric doors that were kept open during the daytime when the weather was good. I favored these doorway areas as pleasant places to sit and look out into the inner square, out onto the roadway encircling the hospital, as well as the surrounding area beyond. As I gazed far off into the disappearing distance I almost felt a part of the open world outside, lost in its expansive space and free of the confining walls of the hospital.

XI. I Am Not Alone

I could immediately see that in this hospital I was not alone in my misfortune. Here, I was similar to everyone else. There were some who were a lot better off than me and some who were a lot worse, which left me somewhere in between. I felt more at ease here, because now I could identify with the other patients around me. In the hospitals in Buffalo I was like a mutant. Compared with my condition, I would have given anything to have been like so many of the patients there. I envied their causes of hospitalization. They were able to get up and walk around, do things for themselves, and in most cases be in and out of the hospital in a matter of a few days. There, in the midst of many, I was alone—not so much physically, but tremendously so psychologically.

Here at West Haverstraw, the patients on my ward ranged in age from mid-teens to the thirties, with one exception being a man appearing to be somewhere in his fifties. Our common lot was that nearly all of us had been healthy and walking about one moment and physically incapacitated the next. Everyone presently found himself confined to a bed, gurney or wheelchair, with no assurance as to just how long.

Most of the injuries were spinal cord injuries resulting from motor vehicle and diving accidents, which were about fifty-fifty. The remaining spinal cord injuries involved knife and gunshot wounds, falls and tumor.

There was one patient, a young guy named Sam, who had not suffered a spinal cord injury but rather lost a leg after being shot by someone he thought wouldn't have the nerve to shoot him. Sam said, "Go ahead and shoot me," and the person actually did. Sam was pretty surprised. To some, Sam might have been thought of as having the type of personality that would have eventually caused someone to shoot him, but I think daring somebody to do it may have been too much of a gamble.

Bearded lumberjack John, who with his facial hair looked a bit like Abraham Lincoln, was a patient whose cubicle was directly across the aisle from mine. He had been among a carload of people when their vehicle went airborne off an embankment and plummeted into a creek below. John found himself outside the car lying in the creek, with an injured neck and neurological damage.

John was somewhat touchy, but an okay guy once one got to know him. He seemed sensitive about his limited education, which did not include completion of high school. On my first day at the hospital I was in my cubicle reading a book and to get my attention John yelled over to me, "Hey smarty!"

One morning John asked Jenny, the meal server, if he could have some scrambled eggs. Jenny told him no, because she thought there were just enough to go to the people who ordered them beforehand. John was upset, but after serving the others Jenny returned with some leftover scrambled eggs. Now John wouldn't accept them, so Jenny just set the plate of eggs on his bed beside him anyway and started to walk away. John said, "Here's your eggs!" and dumped them plate and all on the floor. I looked over at John and his resemblance to Abe Lincoln began to fade. Difficult circumstances or not, would "Honest Abe" ever have felt justified in throwing eggs on the floor?

With physical therapy John eventually regained the ability to walk with the aid of a single metal crutch consisting of a pole, hand grip and arm support band, but his hand and arm function remained affected. While in one of the physical therapy rooms one afternoon, I looked up and saw John go walking past in the corridor pushing his empty wheelchair. I remarked to myself, "Wow, he's actually walking!" and thought it would be great to be able to get to that stage myself. However, the effects of spinal cord injury vary greatly from case to case and John was one of the more fortunate persons.

The sad thing about John was that he had no family for support and was lacking in education. He had been a lumberjack in the Northern woods and had no other vocation. When the time for his discharge from the hospital came John told everyone he was going to a halfway house, but where he really was headed was a nursing home. How different it might have been if only he had a family, an education, or both.

Seeing how similar I was to the other patients around me, it was not surprising that I felt quite at home at West Haverstraw. The entire hospital program was focused on evaluating and dealing with conditions having specific physical limitations, in our cases on Ward A&B, a damaged central nervous system with accompanying effects on normal sensory and motor function.

The goal of the hospital was to adequately respond to every aspect of patient needs. Treatment went beyond physical rehabilitation alone and extended to rehabilitation of the total person. So, there were activities and services in the psychological, educational, vocational, recreational, religious, social and cultural areas as well. The strategy was to meet the heart of the rehabilitation challenge head-on, focusing heavily on the main and necessary areas of concern and encompassing any further needs that might exist. The final objective was to develop to the fullest extent the present capabilities and potential of each individual patient.

I underwent a series of extensive physical examinations and evaluations during my first few days at the hospital. These included blood tests, bladder and kidney examination, X-rays, electrocardiogram, respiratory capacity test, dental examination and general checkup. The results of these evaluations were combined with muscle and range of motion tests done by the physical and occupational therapy departments to provide a point of reference from which to direct a rehabilitation plan. Also, I met with a hospital psychologist for personality and scholastic aptitude testing, a social worker to discuss financial and other matters, and consulted with a vocational rehabilitation counselor to discuss educational opportunities.

Periodically, all persons involved with my rehabilitation program met to discuss the status, progress and future direction of rehabilitation treatment. As with every patient, a final conference that included my family would eventually be held when it was time for me to be released from the hospital. In this way the proper transfer from hospital to home could be discussed and arranged, and future progress and integration into the environment outside the hospital analyzed. It all involved a complex and coordinated effort on the part of many different individuals.

My therapy treatments consisted of four 30-minute physical therapy sessions and one 30-minute occupational therapy session Monday through Friday. Daily physical therapy sessions were: 30 minutes of standing on a "tilt table" that could be adjusted to any angle up to 90 degrees; 30 minutes in a Hubbard tank (whirlpool bath) or in the hospital swimming pool; 30 minutes of ADL (activities of daily living) work with an assigned therapist; 30 minutes of mat work, work with weights, or resistive muscle exercises and passive range of motion exercises, again with the assistance of a therapist or student therapist.

Ann, young and with a freckled face framed by short brown hair, was one of my first physical therapists. While on the tilt table one day it was raised at too much of a vertical angle for me to tolerate. Ann was lost in her thoughts, planning a home-cooked dinner of fried chicken for her parents who were coming to West Haverstraw from out of town. In trying to decide how many pieces of chicken to prepare Ann used me as a measuring stick, asking "How many pieces of chicken could you eat, Ron?" By this time I was about ready to pass out on the tilt table. Ann noticed when I didn't respond to the chicken question and quickly lowered the table. But by then I was too queasy and light-headed to want anything at all to do with fried chicken, so Ann got no help from me.

My occupational therapy sessions consisted of practicing typing, writing, hair grooming, shaving, teeth brushing, washing, using dinner utensils and learning how to use arm and shoulder muscles in the most efficient manner.

For the remaining part of each day I was free do whatever I wanted, provided I was not scheduled for a consultation or some other appointment. During this time I usually did such things as visit with other patients or hospital personnel, wheel randomly about the hospital, watch television, or read. Often I gathered with a group of patients at a lobby near some vending machines just down the corridor from our ward, drinking coffee and talking the time away. Evenings I occasionally attended a movie, bingo game, party, or one of the other recreational activities that were a regular or spur-of-the-moment part of the recreation program at the hospital.

For those patients in satisfactory physical condition, time away from the hospital was allowed by weekend passes covering from after working day on Friday until Sunday night. Or, patients could sign out for any part of a weekend, or even during weekday nights as long as they reported back to the hospital by curfew time. Since I frequently had visitors on weekends, I often took advantage of these opportunities.

One weekend before summer ended, I ventured with family north along the Hudson River on winding Route 9W past Bear Mountain State Park and on up to historical West Point military academy with its impressive scenic setting. We then came back to cross the Hudson at Bear Mountain Bridge and traveled south along the east bank of the river. We drove past Sing Sing prison in Ossining and on through North Tarrytown into the legendary area of Washington Irving's Sleepy Hollow. At Tarrytown we again crossed the spanning Hudson by way of the Tappan Zee Bridge over to Nyack south of West Haverstraw, and from there followed 9W back to the hospital.

On another summer weekend the town of Haverstraw, located right on the riverfront just a bit southeast of West Haverstraw, held a large parade that I attended, again with family members. As bands passed by under the bright blue canopy of a perfect mid-summer day, rich vibrant hues of Revolutionary uniforms flooded my visual senses as rousing sounds of patriotic fife and drum tunes accentuated the steps of hundreds of marching feet. While penetrating rays of sunshine warmed the whole of my inner being I let my mind be carried away to another place and time, completely obliterating my awareness that before long I would be resuming my role as hospital patient.

And when such weekends were over I would indeed once more find myself back at the rehab center assuming the same daily routine as the other patients there, many of whom did not have the chance to get out on weekends.

Alex was a paraplegic patient on Ward A&B who spent almost all of his time laying on his stomach on a gurney. One time when he did get into a wheelchair he looked so different that at first it was hard to believe it was Alex. Alex moved his gurney about with the use of two rubber-tipped canes. His agility with the canes was so good that one day when someone dropped a quarter near the vending machines Alex offered, "I'll get it." Darned if he didn't pick the quarter right up off the floor with his canes!

Alex had powerful arms and was the only one who could easily handle the service roadway hill outside Ward A&B on a gurney. Another paraplegic patient on our ward, Terry, wanted to get to the picnic area one day and tried going down the hill on a gurney. Bad decision. He lost control of the gurney, ran off the road and flipped. Luckily, Terry landed in deep, soft grass and hurt nothing but his pride.

Some of the paraplegic patients really built up their arms in physical therapy. That became clear when the paraplegic guy in the cubicle next to me called out asking to borrow a record from the person in the cubicle on the other side of me. The guy with the record yelled a return warning to get ready to catch it, then sailed the disk like a Frisbee overhead through the air past my cubicle. The record made it to the target cubicle but didn't quite clear the tall clothes locker sitting against the cubicle partition, so the record landed on top of it. I thought to myself, "nice try," and figured that was the end of that. All of a sudden I heard a commotion and looked up to see this guy dragging himself up the partition until he reached the record. "You've got to be kidding!" was my next thought. He must have wanted that record very badly.

John, a college student from Tonawanda, a suburb of Buffalo, had been attending the University of Nebraska. While traveling across the Midwest plains with a group of guys in an open-top MG, the car flipped and crashed, breaking John's neck and leaving him with spinal cord injury quadriplegia. John came to West Haverstraw for rehabilitation, but now was homesick because he was so family and friend-oriented. His family began making arrangements to have John transferred to the same hospital I left to come to West Haverstraw. I told John and his family of my experience with and feelings about that hospital, but John transferred there anyway to be closer to family and friends.

Fifteen-year-old Robin from Syracuse was quite a character. He was a big guy with dark curly hair and a good sense of humor considering his predicament. Robin had dived into shallow water and injured his neck at a high level, so he didn't have much functional capability. Robin zoomed around in a bright orange, upholstered electric wheelchair, and attached to it was a lap board upon which generally could be found a reel-to-reel tape recorder.

Robin's signature behavior was stopping alongside an electrical outlet in a deserted stretch of the main hospital corridor, having someone plug in the tape recorder, and rocking out. To find him one simply followed such tunes blasting through the corridors as Steppenwolf's "Magic Carpet Ride," Cream's "White Room," Creedence Clearwater Revival's "Proud Mary," or the Rolling Stones' "Honky Tonk Woman."

One day Robin had to spend the day in bed, so he urged me to try using his wheelchair. Usually I was very much against electric wheelchairs, because I wanted the physical activity of using a manual one. Yet, on this particular day I decided it might be interesting to see the difference.

I got into Robin's chair and buzzed down to the physical therapy department. There was a new student there, and I couldn't resist having some fun with her. I told her I had just gotten a new electric wheelchair but was not yet very good at driving it. She offered to set up an obstacle course and see how I maneuvered through it. Once it was set up I started through the course, but didn't try to be careful at all. I rammed into one of the course-markers and exclaimed, "Oops!" then shoved the chair into reverse and ran over another. When I turned a corner I plowed through a whole string of them. The student couldn't believe how badly I was doing. One of my regular therapists noticed what was going on and came over to say shame on me. More like mercy on me, because the student was about to kill me!

Robin was quite smitten with one of my physical therapists, Toni, and showed up during my therapy sessions with her to tell her she had million dollar legs. I could put up with only so much of that before chasing him away. Robin could admire and compliment Toni's legs later; my therapy time was important.

Still, I felt bad for Robin. He told me he would never have the chance to experience a normal, intimate guy-girl relationship and wondered what that would be like. It was something that really bothered him. And I understood, because the incomparable high radiating from the total spectrum of such a true and close bond can be among the most wonderful and fulfilling of experiences. The younger a person is when spinal cord injury occurs, the more is lost out on in life.

On weekends Robin's father would arrive at West Haverstraw in his blazing red Corvette to spend time with his son. I often accompanied him as he walked the hospital corridors, and we always talked about Robin. He felt so badly about his son's injury. Parents suffer greatly seeing their children in such difficult situations, and I could clearly sense the tremendous pain Robin's father was feeling.

Limited in immediate travel to wheelchairs and not having cars at hand, patients could not readily leave the grounds and go wherever they wanted when feeling the impulse to the escape the hospital setting and gain the freedom of being away for a while in the ordinary outside world. At times a need for this was felt. Lacking a wide array of choices, there was but a single haven within a mile of the hospital grounds that could be traveled to by wheelchair when seeking a nearby, accessible refuge to which to get away for a while. This was the Fife and Drum—a pub whose name reflected the proud history of its locale—nestled at the end of a gently sloping roadway that served as a back entrance to and exit from the hospital grounds.

There was a very steep hill to the front of the hospital leading down to busy Route 9W, but to the rear the immediately surrounding area was fairly level, at least enough so that the road leading from the hospital and continuing down to the Fife and Drum could be successfully traveled by wheelchair. Since this road was downhill most of the way, getting to the Fife and Drum was easy. When returning, there was a choice of either wheeling back to the hospital or taking a taxi. If patients signed out toward evening to leave the grounds by wheelchair, they were strongly advised to always take a cab back to the hospital instead of wheeling back in the dark.

At times some of the guys on our ward would get adventurous and set out for the Fife and Drum. Although my paraplegic buddies with their much stronger arms offered to help me along the road there and back, I preferred going when having visitors with me to assist in traveling the sloping grade, the incline of which steepened near its town-side end, and as social companions too while there. The Fife and Drum served as a nearby place to go to spend time in a different atmosphere than the hospital. Once relaxed inside, the reward of music, games, snacks and liquid refreshments, and socializing made the effort of journeying there and back worthwhile.

One night two guys from Ward A&B, both named Terry—one of them being the Terry of the infamous gurney-flipping episode—were wheeling back from the Fife and Drum after dark and were nearing the hospital grounds. Being paraplegic, they both had good arm function and could wheel up the sloping grade from the pub without much problem. However, a car approached from behind at a point in the road where it had to come around a curve before being able to see the two wheelers. Worried about his safety, the gurney-flipping Terry moved closer to the edge of the road so he won't be run over.

The road was narrow and there wasn't much of a shoulder at all, but rather an immediate drop-off into an adjoining field. Like the

70

gurney crash revisited, Terry dropped off the edge, turning over the wheelchair and being dumped out into the field as he toppled over. With the help of the surviving Terry, he managed to get back into his wheelchair and up onto the road again, and since he wasn't hurt they both returned laughing about the whole affair.

Since biblical times beverages bearing an alcohol content—most notably wine beginning back then—have been strongly ingrained in cultural tradition. They became staples of everyday living throughout various parts of the world. In moderation drinks containing alcohol have been quite socially acceptable, and in limitation in a positive and prudent manner unwanted effects do not accompany their use. Yet varieties of such beverages have widely multiplied, and when used in excess or for the wrong reason problems can swiftly arise. As a means of escape, coping, or simply pursuing the feeling of intoxication alcoholic beverages have no positive qualities.

Alcohol was not allowed on hospital grounds, though almost always some patient could be found in possession of some form of it, especially on weekends. At times there was excessive on-grounds consumption, and as a result of behavior in their inhibition-freeing condition the imbibers would be discovered and then found themselves in serious trouble.

Luckily such goings-on weren't common, but on my very first night at the hospital a few guys drank too much Southern Comfort whiskey and one of them got violent and started breaking up the place. Although very powerful he was subdued, restrained and finally sedated, because even though the staff managed to get him into bed he still attempted out of sheer frustration to put his fist through the thick glass partition of his cubicle wall. Even though everyone involved was almost booted out of the hospital right then and there, on this occasion no one actually left. However, when following repeat offenses occurred, expulsions from the hospital were carried out.

In a much less serious episode, Terry, who had already had the gurney and wheelchair mishaps, returned to the ward late one night after being out drinking. He came flying through the entrance to A wing where his cubicle was located, but there was a CircOlectric bed in the first cubicle that stuck out a bit into the aisle. Terry hit the bed and his body whipped forward at the waist, even though he managed to stay in the chair this time. However, he had a pint of whiskey hidden inside his shirt and as he went forward the bottle flew out and skidded down the middle of the aisle with a loud clatter. Terry was a good-natured guy, and alcohol usually just put him in a happier mood if anything. So, he ended up with only a stern lecture, confiscation of the whiskey, and an immediate trip to bed.

The alcohol use that did take place usually didn't cause serious problems. Most patients didn't make a habit of abusing it, so the staff often looked the other way and there were those who even helped obtain it. For some patients it was just another recreational pastime along with the other more legitimate activities at the hospital.

This is not in any way a defense or approval of alcohol use, but merely an observation of it as part of the behavior of a number of the hospital patients. Without the right frame of mind and respect for the influence on behavior it can have, improper use of alcohol can have unwanted consequences and become too easy to fall into a pattern of abuse. The biblical warning that whoever is lead astray by drink is not wise (Proverbs 20:1) holds great truth and an indispensable lesson to be applied in everyday living.

Harry was a 16-year-old paraplegic patient on Ward A&B injured during the winter when the sled he was riding downhill continued into the road in front of an oncoming vehicle. His father thought it was a stupid thing for Harry to have done, and didn't seem too sympathetic with Harry's plight. In fact, he seemed more angry than sympathetic.

Harry wasn't very popular, and many people even made fun of him. Whatever his appearance and personality were, he still was faced with the same tough situation as the rest of us on the ward. Everyone was different in his own way, and Harry certainly couldn't be faulted for that.

One weekend some of Harry's family, including his father, arrived on the ward to visit. While some of the others were with Harry, his father strolled over to my cubicle to talk with me. He was holding a bag of potato chips and offered some to me. I told him "No, thanks," since I really didn't want any of the chips. But even if I did want some I wouldn't have taken them, because I was lying flat on my back in bed and would have had a hard time eating them in that position.

Paying no attention at all to what I had just said, Harry's father dumped some potato chips onto my chest, telling me "Come on, have some!" I just ignored the chips, and when he realized it might be hard for me to eat them in my position in bed, Harry's father said "Oh, I forgot," as he started shoving some of the chips into my mouth. I still didn't want them, but figured I might as well eat the few that were there just to satisfy him.

As I was forcing down the chips he next came out with, "I guess you're going to have a long time to think about this," as he nodded his head in a motioning direction toward my body. He was referring to my accident and its accompanying consequences.

From this statement and the way he said it I assumed that what he really meant was something like, "Well, you got what you deserved; maybe this will teach you a lesson!"

Instantly I snapped back defensively with, "What's there to think about? An accident's an accident!"

Actually, what Harry's father said was true. I just didn't agree with his seemingly uncaring "You asked for it, now live with it" attitude toward me, Harry, or anybody on our ward. Sure, I'd have a long time to think about what my mistake cost me. I knew that better than he or anyone else.

I was painfully aware that my accident was a direct result of not living my life as wisely and maturely as I could have, and knew I would continue thinking about that every day of my life. The saying, "The truth hurts," is accurate and that's what bothered me more than anything. Still, it would have been better to not have Harry's father insensitively reminding people of their follies just because he was right and felt his point should be made. I was way ahead of him in realizing I had largely woven my own fate.

It would have been easy to use the excuse that icy roads, poor traction of my auto's light back end, not letting Ray drive home instead of me, or any combination of things, caused the accident that resulted in my life-altering spinal cord injury. The inescapable fact, though, was that in an irresponsible and irreversible way I simply made wrong decisions that night. I had the repeated chance that evening to make a much smarter choice and be in a different and safe place where I really wanted to be, yet didn't do it. Not being strong enough to do what I wanted and should have done cost me in an unrecoverable way and changed the entire future course of my life.

After actor Yul Brenner died of lung cancer a posthumous American Cancer Society TV commercial showed him saying, "If I could take back that smoking we wouldn't be talking about any cancer, I'm convinced of that." Well, if I could take back the irresponsibility of driving after a night of continued social drinking we wouldn't be talking about any spinal cord injury, I'm convinced of that. A lot of people would no doubt like to go back and correct past errors in judgment, but in life major mistakes have to be avoided before they occur because that's when the correct decisions have to be made. Once something happens that has unwanted consequences, there isn't a second chance to go back and do things the right way.

At least Brenner made it through his youthful years unscathed, but his testimony brings to light how unwise and self-destructive human behavior can sometimes be. People at times tend to not face their true vulnerability until it is right upon them. By then whatever might have happened may not be easy to correct, if it even can be corrected. All too often we do not want to admit we are mortal and vulnerable beings, and because of this the God-given health and well-being we start off with is not as appreciated and protected as it should be.

Harry's father wore a brace on one leg, possibly as the result of contracting polio when he was younger. If this was the case then his cynical attitude toward spinal cord injury victims, mostly young males whose risk-taking behavior played a primary role in their injury, might be at least somewhat understandable. He may have figured that while his affliction was something over which he had no control, we were foolish agents of our own misfortune so we essentially got what we deserved. I'm not sure just how constructive such an attitude is, even if there was a measure of truth in it.

Yet, I think luck also is a factor in unfortunate events. I had friends who had worse accidents than mine and escaped virtually unharmed. For instance, a short while before my accident one friend flipped his Chevelle Super Sport end-over-end at a high rate of speed. The tire jack in the trunk flew right past his head and through the windshield, barely missing him. But, there he was the following night sitting next to me telling me about it and having not much more than a lot of soreness.

Another acquaintance had a bad accident and ended up lying in the road in the middle of an intersection. He also escaped serious injury. And, of course, Ray was uninjured while with me at the time of my accident. So fate sometimes strikes in an unpredictable way at a given time and there's no way to foresee and prevent that except perhaps for more cautious and sensible living, which many younger people seem unable to do. Surely youth is a wonderful time to enjoy life, if a person's well-being is not sacrificed in the process.

A couple of historic events occurred while I was at West Haverstraw during the summer of '69. The first was the moon landing by U.S. astronauts, which I watched on TV with awe. If modern technology could send men to the moon, why couldn't it be used to cure spinal cord injury?

The second event was Woodstock, which took place not far north of West Haverstraw. I might have attended Woodstock had I not gotten injured, because that was the type of thing I was apt to do at the stage in life I was at. That weekend the daytime ward head nurse, Marie, went to Woodstock. On Monday she reported to me that there were people everywhere and lots of mud because of rain. She said the music was good, the parking wasn't, and that someone lying on the ground in a sleeping bag was run over. Still, Marie said that overall she had a good time. Being so close I wished I could have been there myself, but the way things were the best I could do was hear about it secondhand.

Sixteen-year-old Joey was a paraplegic patient who also had drug dependency and suicidal risk problems. Each night he tried to get injections of the pain-relieving drug Demerol from the nurses. If they didn't give him what he wanted when he wanted it he would slam his fist against the thick glass of his cubicle partition and say, "You'd better read what's on my chart!" On it, of course, was the suicidal tendency notation.

Eye-catching hospital volunteer, Gloria, who rode a motorcycle and looked great in black leather, tried to influence Joey for the better. That would have worked for me and I'd have probably asked her to get a sidecar. But Joey was more interested in drugs than in attractive women and good intentions, and failed to respond to Gloria's mission. If we wanted to talk further about wrong decisions, all that needed to be said to validate the seriousness of their impact was that Joey died of a drug overdose after leaving the hospital.

One person who impressed me was an ex-patient named John. John's condition was quadriplegia, but he was a determined overachiever who functioned like someone with paraplegia. John was completely independent and, driving there himself, had returned to the hospital to be readmitted for a brief checkup. He could transfer to and from car and bed, dress himself, and wheel his chair with almost paraplegic ease.

In talking to him about my rehabilitation progress I made the statement, "I'd like to be where you are."

John replied, "You'll get there."

Functional improvement can eventually come in spinal cord injury, but it takes time. A bit of determination and effort doesn't hurt either. In John's case a physical therapist took a special interest in him, and the result was his high achievement.

There was someone I had known for several years who I had grown quite close to in the last two years before my accident. During my stays at the hospitals in Buffalo in the first half of '69, Joyce was in Kansas City training to be a flight attendant so I didn't see that much of her. To be able to see me more often, she switched to working as a photographer for a national photo group. By the time I was ready to go to West Haverstraw, Joyce had gotten assigned to that area. Thinking I would already be in West Haverstraw, she showed up at the hospital the weekend before I arrived.

When I got to West Haverstraw I right away became friends with the gurney and wheelchair-flipping Terry from A wing of Ward A&B. Terry was from Watertown, New York up near the St. Lawrence River, and was at the rehab center because of the spinal cord injury that occurred when his back was broken in a dump truck accident. It was Terry who told me someone had been at the hospital the previous weekend looking for me. From the description he gave, I knew it was Joyce.

In the year of my accident the bond between us grew to the point where it could have become permanent. Sincere of heart and fully devoted, Joyce was ready but I wasn't as mature or settled so it remained uncertain just where our relationship was headed. I wanted to continue having Joyce in my life, yet on terms more suitable to my needs than hers. Joyce was special and important to me, so within me was the potential to completely and unconditionally commit to her. Yet until I was ready to give that commitment, what existed between us had only sand castle stability.

Still, my feeling of natural closeness to her meant my relationship with Joyce would go forward in whatever unknown direction it was headed, with time and the easing of my inner unsettledness being its strongest allies. This depended, though, on no catastrophic life changes such as a car accident resulting in spinal cord injury. Enough pre-injury uncertainties already existed. It would be a stretch to add dramatic, post-injury changes and not expect them to seriously destabilize the future course of our relationship.

XII. A Special Interest

I like the way you walk,
I like the way you talk,
Susie Q.

Lyrics from "Susie Q"
Creedence Clearwater Revival

Sometimes when there is need for an extra ray of light a shining
star appears, radiating bright beams of encouragement and uplifting
hope and spirit. Although I was determined to overcome on my own
the challenges facing me, an important boost to the positive attitude
that helped fuel my rehabilitation goals was the presence and special
interest of a nurse's aide at the hospital in Buffalo before I transferred
to West Haverstraw.

A raven-haired beauty of slender feminine form that very well
complemented the soft blue uniform dress she wore, 18-year-old Sue
was friendly and outgoing and had a great sense of humor. I took an
immediate liking to her and before long it became clear that she had
taken more than an ordinary interest in me. My roommate made a
simple but true observation when Sue left the room after spending
time with me one night—"She likes you."

Sue's entire demeanor had as much effect on me as her
captivating looks. I could feel the magnetic draw of her mere
presence, even though in my outward behavior I dared not be
presumptuous enough to assume we might be anything more to each
other than that defined by our patient-nurse's aide roles. My reality
was that I could no longer freely act on inner impulses and desires. I

had lost both self-value and confidence as a male having interest in a female, and was not readily going to take rejection risks in opposite sex relations.

Still, I couldn't help naturally responding to Sue. One thing making interaction with her easier was that she worked the 3 to 11 P.M. shift, when floor supervision was less strict. The young attractive blonde nurse in charge on this shift, Debbie, was Sue's close friend. Debbie was fun-loving, not the serious type at all, and she and Sue joked around quite a bit and really had a time. Yet, they were efficient and did their duties well when these had to be done.

On the night of my birthday, March 17, Sue and Debbie paraded into my room holding high a flaming cake and singing "Happy Birthday." Turning 23 in the hospital wasn't the way I wanted things to be, but at least someone was focusing on it positively.

Sue would usually have me assigned as one of her patients whenever she was on duty, and she spent a lot of time with me. If she had weekends off, she sometimes would come to the hospital to take me for a walk either inside the building or outside somewhere. Our mutual attraction continued to grow, blossoming into an unspoken bond reinforced by the daily presence of each other. Yet, neither of us openly admitted that there was anything between us. Our budding relationship was just something that gradually developed and then was suddenly there without deliberately pursuing it.

During the first part of my stay at the hospital in Buffalo Sue had a boyfriend, but their relationship began to deteriorate and eventually ended. I was involved with Joyce at the time of my accident, but my way of thinking about her had changed because I found it so difficult relating to her the way things now were. There simply was too much difference between the before and after images of our relationship, and I was having a hard time trying to resolve that.

My closeness with Sue came from her knowledge of what I presently was, and her ease in accepting and dealing with that in all of her interactions with me. She was right there much of the time, and was an important part of my hospital care. Sue saw me struggle during the early rough times, and seemed to know what I was going through and what having my type of injury meant. Because she had such close knowledge of me and seeing my shortcomings still held me in special regard, Sue had a much easier entrance than anyone else through the gate of my post-injury defenses. She was the one person with whom I was somewhat at ease and to whom I was always receptive.

With hard-to-accept contradictions flooding my mind, Sue provided a much needed "time out" from dwelling on the down side of things. As I focused my thoughts on her, she became a comforting refuge from an otherwise very disheartening life situation.

On her nineteenth birthday in June, Sue was surprised to receive a dozen long-stemmed, red roses. She wasn't surprised by the name "Caesar" on the card, because it was her pet name for me. She had come to work one afternoon and walked into my room. There I was sitting high in my CircOlectric bed with the back raised almost straight up. Sue remarked, "You look just like Caesar sitting on his throne!"

Whether or not I in any way resembled Caesar on his throne was debatable. What was clear was I didn't have his power and control to change things by simple command. If I did, I'd command my spinal cord to heal itself and free me from the "throne" upon which I now sat.

Getting the roses emotionally moved Sue and drew her even closer to me. Yet the growing ties between us were about to be disrupted, because soon I would be leaving for West Haverstraw. Although I felt a strong attraction to Sue, my thoughts were focused heavily on the rehabilitation opportunities awaiting me there. I thought once I left Buffalo Sue probably would not continue to be much more than a very pleasant memory. She was the one thing in Buffalo I didn't want to leave behind, but I needed to move on with my forward progress.

It would not end that easily. Shortly after my arrival at West Haverstraw writing became one of the activities of my occupational therapy program, so we kept in contact through the mail. Sue also telephoned to keep in touch that way. The connection between us was a long way from being broken.

Having been at West Haverstraw for three months, it was now October. It was a colorful and picturesque time of the year in the Hudson River Valley, but natural beauty suddenly showed up in another form. Sue had planned a surprise trip to West Haverstraw and arrived for a few days visit. What would happen now? Clearly something had developed between us, but separation had kept it limited. With her increased presence Joyce had re-entered the picture, and without Sue around I had been accepting her as well as my uncertain psychological state allowed.

Sue's arrival turned potential into reality, because what existed under the surface now had the opportunity to expand into an open and acknowledged thing. Sue knew my injury had dramatically changed whatever relationship I had with Joyce, and also knew it was she herself who I was very accepting of, felt comfortable with, and easily related to. So, it wasn't hard to assume she likely would have success if she wanted to openly establish something between us.

After driving all day from Buffalo, about an 8-hour trip, Sue pulled into West Haverstraw on a Thursday evening. Exhausted from the drive, she stayed only a short while at the hospital before leaving to spend the night at the Holiday Inn Hotel in New City, a few miles south of West Haverstraw. As she left, I told Sue I would try to find housing for her at or near the hospital so she wouldn't have to stay in a motel.

The next day I asked one of my physical therapists, Sheila, if she knew a place where Sue might stay. With perfect timing, Sheila was leaving town later in the day and said Sue could stay at her apartment while she was away. Before leaving the hospital, Sheila stopped by the ward and dropped off a key.

While I was busy with my daily schedule of therapy, Sue spent much of Friday catching up on her rest. By the time she showed up at the hospital in the evening, she was pretty much recuperated from the previous day's ordeal. I had the apartment key for her, and that perked her up even more.

Not knowing in time about Sue's visit, I told her about previous plans I had made with the two Terry's from Ward A&B to go to a night spot in Spring Valley, located south of West Haverstraw beyond New City, Saturday evening. I explained that we had reservations at the Spring Valley Holiday Inn and were going to stay there overnight. There were going to be aides from the hospital at the nightclub to give whatever assistance was needed at the hotel afterward, and between their help and that of the Terry's things appeared in good shape and I was looking forward to this outing. Sue asked if she could come along and I said sure, I didn't think the guys would mind. Besides, with Sue along I wouldn't need help from anyone else because she surely would be in good control of things.

Saturday afternoon, onto the ward strode Sue wearing a richly-hued, crimson blouse that formed a perfect buffer between her raven-colored hair and jet black miniskirt. Instantly drawing the attention of Syracuse rockin' Robin, the look on his face told me he was likely re-evaluating the status he had assigned to my physical therapist Toni as holder of the Miss Million Dollar Legs title.

Robin's cubicle was kitty-corner to mine across the aisle, and when Sue knelt down to help me put on a pair of dress shoes I was thought he was going to fall right out of his wheelchair. Robin was still an adolescent, and all it took was something like the flash of a halfway decent pair of female legs to set him off. In Sue's case, the long shapely legs she was showing far exceeded a halfway decent rating.

Setting out for Spring Valley, Sue and I drove south along the Hudson on scenic Route 9W in her little tan Chevy Corvair while the two Terry's took a taxi. Not too far out of Haverstraw Sue pulled into a roadside parking area overlooking the river and we talked for a while. The concession truck that sold the best hot dogs with sauerkraut around was there as usual doing a booming business.

Sue projected a strong feminine presence, and one with which she was very much in touch. I could feel its effect, and sitting next to her with an inescapable full view of her well-sculpted legs it was obvious that Sue was indeed a threat to Toni's Robin-assigned million dollar legs title. For me, though, it was nice just being with Sue away from the hospital. Yet, internally I was not completely content because of a storm of conflicting emotions. It was great being together, but agony wondering if I could really have her as a girlfriend with the physical limitations I had. I felt out of place, not as much as I had with Joyce, but still it was hard seeing what she was physically and then looking at myself. It had never been this way in my pre-injury life. I wanted to react to Sue on her level without restrictions, but there were too many shackles around me to have the relationship with her I really wanted.

At Holiday Inn we checked into two rooms, one for the Terry's and the other for me and Sue. No longer could there be pretending or denial. This night together would surely bring to the surface whatever there was between us. And if a relationship did truly exist, the private time we were about to share would spawn an awareness that it should be openly acknowledged and further developed if that was what was meant to be.

As evening approached the guys were excited about going to the nightclub, saying they were going to drink, listen to music and dance in their wheelchairs. Despite their prodding, Sue and I decided to stay at the motel. We didn't feel we would miss much by not going out, because all we really wanted was to spend some time by ourselves. We talked, lounged around and watched TV, and then Sue left the room to take a shower and get ready for bed.

Alone with my thoughts while Sue was out of the room, I suddenly realized this was not fantasy—I really was going to be alone with her the whole night. Wanting so much to have Sue with me my anticipation was soaring, yet at the same time it all seemed somehow spoiled because physically I was a long way from being what I wanted to and felt I should be once again. Sue was the support I needed, but my inner confusion remained a serious concern.

When it started, the gush of the shower seized my attention and seemed to draw me right into the stall with Sue. It was an inviting, almost hypnotic sound that brought delightful visions of Sue standing majestically amidst forceful streams with torrents of spray cascading over her shapely form. Yet, this intoxicating high instantly turned to nervous uncertainty when the hiss of the spray suddenly stopped.

I suffered through what seemed an eternity of silence before the bathroom door swung open. Out strutted Sue wearing a short, lace-trimmed white chiffon nightie—a sight that at once quickened my breath and heartbeat—and stood before me in well-deserved female pride before unhesitatingly sliding into bed beside me.

It was a visual feast taking in the view of Sue before she got into bed. Lying so closely beside me, her feminine allure overwhelmed me and before long we were kissing and embracing. Although Sue's receptiveness was encouraging, this would be a night of limited closeness because my physical restrictions meant that my initiative would be restrained no matter how appealing Sue was. And this also was our first time alone together, so we were going to let our comfort with each other develop at its own pace.

With just the spoken expression of my feelings, I could have unlocked much within Sue's heart. I could have communicated my need for her in words that do not fail to evoke response in a woman. Yet I remained silent, largely because of the intense internal war being waged between my attraction to Sue and the doubts I had about my masculine self-image. My self-assurance was affected and a hindrance to expressing myself more openly to her. I had fallen victim to self-doubt instead of overcoming it by directly and honestly communicating to her my innermost thoughts and feelings.

Any further closeness with Sue this night would be in my dreams. Sleep overcame us after just kissing her and holding her in my arms. Still, we had spent time getting to know each other on another level, and that itself was important to our budding relationship.

As the sun rose and daylight filtered gently into the room, I awoke to see Sue asleep beside me in resplendent beauty. Her hair, its lustrous sheen gleaming like fine black pearls, gathered softly to each side of her face on the white background of her pillow. I gazed wistfully at the wondrous vision before me—inviting pink lips, ivory-smooth skin, shapely feminine form from bosom to thighs. In this silent moment I was in complete possession of Sue in a very special and private way, without fear of how my failings might prevent me from having her in the true reality of my world.

Coaxing Sue from her sleep, morning brought with it a noticeable lessening of whatever inhibitions she may have had the night before. Although a welcome overture, something more immediate was putting reins on our growing closeness and comfort with each other. We had a checkout deadline to meet and had to get ready to leave the hotel. As if to verify this, the phone suddenly rang. It was the Terry's, wondering when we would be ready to go.

As we left the hotel and were heading back to West Haverstraw, I began thinking about the time I had just spent with Sue. It was a bittersweet experience of the mountain-peak high of privately basking in her presence and the crevice-deep low of the frustration of not being able to fully respond to her in the way she was making me feel. Yet, the different mood of the morning signaled our relationship's continuing development despite the initial, self-imposed shackling of my responses to Sue.

Sue's receptiveness was there all along, but she was waiting for me to take control as our growing closeness unfolded and by morning realized I needed help. Taking control was the key. If I could do it, it would be a complete change where I focused more on open, spoken communication instead of silent, direct action. Before, I acted out my feelings. Now, I had to verbally communicate them. Sue had shown she was ready to take a more active role in her outward behavior, but was I ready and capable of assuming a role where much of my interaction with her was verbal expression of inner feelings?

Could I overcome my dissatisfaction with my physical status and self-image so I could accept the role I would need to take in my relationship with Sue? Right now I felt victimized and out of control, and was unsure of being able to openly and honestly communicate my inner feelings the way I knew I would need to. I wanted whatever closeness I could have with Sue, but at the same time had concerns about whether I actually was capable of meeting her expectations for the relationship we were forming.

And, there was more to consider. What about Joyce? If Sue hadn't re-entered the picture, would I have eventually stabilized enough psychologically to accept Joyce's wish to continue our relationship? As things now stood Joyce was in a no-win situation against Sue, because Sue was such a refuge of security for me. Yet, was it fair to reject Joyce's continued dedication and turn to someone else?

The answer clearly was no. But my whole world had been turned upside down, and things were so unacceptably different that I was having problems both in facing them and in relating to Joyce. Unless either things returned to the way they were before my accident or I somehow came to terms with all that had happened to me, any relationship between us was going to be difficult.

It was a struggle finding a way to feel comfortable with Joyce in my new identity. I thought back to how we related to one another before, and now for me at least that had completely changed. I felt alienated from Joyce because of how things had so suddenly and dramatically shifted, and was not having much success accepting her willingness to continue our relationship despite her realization that things were very different now from what they were before.

I was not the same person; I had lost too much. My pre-injury, elevated status with Joyce was gone. Maybe she could accept this dramatic devaluation of what I was, but I couldn't. Joyce's lofty image of me had been important, and a central part of our relationship. I couldn't be to her what I was before, and couldn't accept having to relate to her in a diminished way.

And even if I tried, there still was no way Joyce could compete with someone who could deal as easily and naturally with all aspects of my new life as Sue. It just wasn't possible at this point in time. I was going with what I felt most comfortable and secure, and that was Sue. It wasn't right and it wasn't fair, but given what I now faced and my feeling of so much lack of control over my life, it was what I chose. Until I could come to terms with myself the way I would eventually need to, it was going to be very difficult to genuinely and unselfishly meet the needs of anyone but myself. In this regard, I surely had yet a long way to go.

When Joyce realized my relationship with Sue had turned into a serious involvement she approached me, asking how Sue fit into the picture. I couldn't answer that, but knew it had become clear to Joyce that her own relationship with me was seriously threatened. By now she had to be feeling she was losing in her attempt to wring from me some kind of genuine commitment to her in response to the dedication and steadfastness she had continued to show.

Reaching the limit of what she shouldn't have had to endure, Joyce let me know I was not giving the effort needed in our relationship and that she could not keep it going all by herself. Joyce didn't want to give up, because she had been doing okay relating to me. But, my difficulty relating to her and involvement with Sue left little else to do.

Joyce rightfully was frustrated with my not giving anything back in our relationship, and had to let me know that. I did not respond to her challenge, but rather let it become a justification for setting aside for the immediate time what existed between us.

Joyce too had become a victim just by being a part of my life at this time. A sudden twist of fate had snatched from her the influence she previously had on me. Joyce lost her continuing connection to me because when I lost my sense of certainty and security I found myself in completely new territory and in my unstable state could not maintain my orientation toward her. Because I couldn't shed or accept my present physical status, I just didn't have a way of working through things so I could deal with Joyce in the way she wanted, expected and deserved.

Although the sudden and unwanted change in my life caused by my accident had brought with it a lot of confusion and uncertainty I didn't know how to handle, it hadn't been easy for Joyce either. And, much of that had been compounded by my approach to it all. Joyce was powerless to get me to realize that what existed between us had not been lost, and that I just needed to hang in there and give things a chance to improve and work out. That was easier said than done, because my mind just could not reconcile past and present. I needed some kind of refuge to escape to so I wouldn't have to deal with all the harsh realities and contradictions confronting me. Sue was that refuge.

Still, what Joyce was remained undiminished in my eyes and it was unfair to compare her with Sue. Regardless of Sue's importance in my present, destabilized world, Joyce had her own before my accident. Sue was a needed help and inspiration in my new life, but if there was any possible way I could have shed my injury and returned to the hopes and potential of my pre-injury future—of which Joyce was a part—that is what I'd have done since I would then regain the control over my life I had lost and so desperately wanted back. There was no magic, though, so the world I had now was with post-injury Sue.

Yet, I totally rejected my post-injury image, and in truth could relate only to what I was before. If Sue had this high a regard for me now, what would she have thought of me in pre-injury times? I viewed my fall in status as unacceptable, yet Sue seemed to think it hadn't devalued me at all. So, whatever relationship Sue wanted with me she could have, **IF** I was able to give it.

Sue was direct and uncomplicated, and what she wanted was very simple. She wanted a special, meaningful relationship where I would participate as fully and honestly as she, and if I did that then how perfect I was physically was not going to be of great importance. Sue had clear ideas about how she wanted our interaction to be, and it was up me to respond in the way she expected.

Yet, even with my limitations Sue did not discount the importance of the physical part of our relationship. Her feeling was that each partner should participate to the fullest extent that each's emotional and physical standing allowed. So to Sue physical expression was just as important as emotional expression, the only difference being that each partner should acknowledge and be true to what he and she really was at that level. Here was where the trouble would start if there was going to be any, because if I could not accept what I presently was physically, that would spill over into the emotional part of our relationship, making its progress and success questionable.

Because of my own uncertainties, I was thankful for Sue's straightforwardness. My physical status seemed to in no way inhibit her direct way of naturally and freely relating to me, and I almost felt like a regular guy in a normal relationship with a girlfriend once again. If I was in my wheelchair and she felt like sitting on my lap she would do that, and during the times I was in bed she would pull the curtains closed around the cubicle and sit on the bed with me. Regardless of what I thought, Sue did not consider my masculine identity diminished and in her behavior toward me did whatever she could to reinforce within me that feeling.

Sue wasn't about to restrict her feminine expression or accept unnecessarily limited physical interaction in our relationship, especially if it helped me feel more confident and self-accepting. In relating to one another she didn't want me to feel any differently about my self-image than I had before my accident.

The challenge for me was meeting Sue's expectations. For our relationship to work, I would have to overcome my feelings of inadequacy and respond to her in a true and genuine way. Any restrictions and limitations on me would be strictly self-imposed and in direct contradiction to how Sue felt and behaved.

After the weekend, Sue and I saw less of each other because of my rigorous daily schedule. Wanting to have more time by ourselves, Sue suggested spending time overnight away from the hospital. Being alone with her again would surely keep our relationship growing, but I would need permission from the hospital for an overnight pass.

The ward doctor might have approved the pass, because if reestablishing interpersonal relationships and reintegration into the world outside the hospital were ultimate rehabilitation goals, then trial periods away from the rehab center such as Sue wanted could be helpful. Yet, from within my deep well of self-doubt there once again rose the thwarting obstacle of hesitation and uncertainty. Without even checking with my doctor about an overnight pass, I told Sue I didn't think staying away from the hospital overnight was allowed during the week because of scheduled morning activities.

Faced with a repeat of my holding back once more, Sue did not push the issue further. But by now she must have been feeling some frustration, since my continuing passiveness was not a help in strengthening and advancing our relationship. How could I want Sue and reject her at the same time?

My inner conflicts didn't make sense. I was strongly drawn to Sue and wanted her to be part of my post-injury life. Yet in almost a destructive way, at the very same time on the surface I was not openly and honestly showing my need for her. This was risky, because Sue didn't know my inner thoughts and feelings and had to rely only on the way I responded to her in my outward behavior.

Sue was doing her part in trying to keep things going in the direction they needed to go. Giving clear signals as to what she expected, she made it obvious that she wanted me to directly and naturally respond to her as a man responding to a woman special to him, but stopped short of pressing beyond that. After throwing out gestures that were met with hesitation, Sue backed off upon seeing me unsure of just how to react.

Sue tried to get me to put aside doubts, reservations, and confidence-affecting concerns and just respond to our relationship in a very simple and open way that kept me focused on it rather than on other less positive things that could only be self-defeating. She didn't want me projecting concerns about what effect my injury had on my present life into our relationship. I was going to have to leave that kind thinking behind if I expected to have a successful relationship with her or anyone else.

Sue had confidence in both me and our relationship, but I needed to have the same feeling. If I was having trouble doing that then she was right there to help, as long as I was willing to give some effort in overcoming whatever problems I was having.

I was unsure of exactly how to respond to Sue, and did not react the way she likely expected given the cues she was sending my way. I was not actively taking control of things, but simply responding to Sue's actions as the situation went along. I didn't feel fully and strongly in control, and this was causing much uneasiness. I could see I was going to have to keep trying to regain a sense of confidence in and control over things confronting me in my new transformed life, and this included my personal relationships.

My inability to accept my post-injury self had already sabotaged the relationship I had with Joyce, but even though things were easier and more comfortable with Sue it was clear there also were problems to overcome with her. I wanted to go forward with our relationship, because I had attached myself to her and she fit so well as a part of my post-injury life. Still, I was having a hard time dealing with the deep and unsettling feeling of loss of control that had filtered into our relationship from my general outlook toward my life situation as it now stood.

I just was not able to confidently be myself as I had so easily done in my pre-injury life. In a role reversal, I left it to Sue to take charge in defining and shaping our developing relationship patterns. If our relationship was to be firmly established as a real and lasting thing, Sue was going to have to be the one carrying most of the weight in getting us to that point.

All my passive indecision, with its effect on Sue's expectations for the growth of our relationship during her visit, even caused Sue to momentarily hesitate. She sensed the reluctance and uncertainty that I, for whatever reason, was experiencing. Wondering if she was going too fast, Sue expressed her concern about pursuing our relationship too strongly.

I told her she wasn't, yet could not open up enough to further reassure her. The truth was, Sue needed to assume the active role she was taking because I was not able to do the same. I was ready to follow Sue's lead, but couldn't take charge of our relationship myself. Without her efforts, things between us would not have advanced as far as they had. I lacked the confidence and control to strongly pursue as a male is normally expected to do. I had willingness, but Sue with her direct and less inhibited approach was the central force actively making the relationship work. But, was it working? Sue wanted more, and expected me to give my share. I felt comfortable with her assuming an assertive role, because it took the pressure off me. I wanted to deal only with resolving my internal identity conflicts and wanted Sue to take charge of the direction of our relationship patterns. She was an accepted and needed part of my new and uncertain world, and I saw her being as assertive and forward as she wanted as not only desirable but necessary. The question was, would Sue accept my marginal level of giving in our relationship? Within, my feelings for Sue were strongly present yet my inner chaos was a barrier to their free outward expression.

Our differences were that whereas Sue was looking past my injury toward relationship images she saw as having the potential to be, I had not put the competing uncertainties of my injury aside so I could focus on having our relationship become what Sue wanted. Sue's images and expectations were much more unclouded and defined than mine, because unlike me her central focus was on the relationship itself rather than on doubts surrounding my post-injury status. While I struggled with internal uncertainties as I tried to look ahead to how my life would be, Sue's expectations were unburdened.

Toward the end of the week Sue told me it was time for her to return to Buffalo, saying that as soon as she could get her finances and other matters straightened out back home she would return to West Haverstraw and see if she could find a job in the area. Wanting to work as a nurse's aide at the rehab center, she had already inquired about that but was told hospital policy did not permit relationships between employees and patients.

Despite the storm of conflicting forces swirling in my mind, Sue seemed confident in our relationship and approached it in a focused, almost worry-free manner. After she left to return to Buffalo I was told by Alan, the male nurse in charge on the 3 to 11 P.M. shift, that during a talk with Sue she said marriage was something she already was considering as an outcome of our relationship.

Our approaches to our relationship truly were different, not in the sense of wanting it to continue growing, which both of us did, but in thinking of its advancement as having no barriers in its way. Sue assumed I was capable of being a stable, giving partner with inner problems, if any, that I could overcome. I wanted to live up to those expectations, but in reality know it was a far reach.

In the presence of the Terry's the morning following our stay at Holiday Inn, Sue had jokingly referred to getting married, wondering what the head of the rehab wing on which she worked and I had been at the hospital in Buffalo would think of that. She clearly had uncomplicated visions and goals for our relationship, and I did not disapprove but simply had competing concerns that were tugging me in their direction.

It was okay with me for Sue to think about our relationship in any way she wanted. Many thoughts were still her own, and when she was ready to reveal them to me she could. It still all came right back to me passively following Sue's lead. In our relationship she had essentially become the pursuing male and me the accepting female.

While Sue focused on our relationship, my priority was getting as completely rehabilitated as possible. There would be plenty of time later for other things, including marriage, if it came to that. And if it did, it would be because that's what Sue wanted. She remained a necessary part of my post-injury life, and no matter what the state of my inner mind and how much I balked and hesitated, in the end I would respond to our relationship the way she wanted if in the meantime she could put up with all of my indecisive behavior.

XIII. A Problem Develops

To act against one's conscience
is neither safe nor honorable.

—Martin Luther

One of my distinguishing characteristics, which at times was an asset and other times not, was that I was not a yes-man. What I did was done my way according to what I thought served me best. I was not impressed by authority or expertise if I thought it was self-serving or did not fully take into account my interests, needs and concerns. This was clear in my earlier transfer to West Haverstraw from the hospital in Buffalo. Yet, there were times when doing things my own hardheaded way brought about disaster, such as the fateful night Ray and I ventured out despite strong advice against doing so.

Nonetheless, for better or worse I made my own decisions and lived with the consequences. Some decisions were right and some wrong. Naturally, I regretted the wrong decisions but accepted responsibility for them and went on from there. Likewise, I felt good about the right decisions and was glad I pursued them with will and determination. I was impulsive and a risk taker, and did not hesitate to take chances when opportunities were at hand. I was spontaneous and unpredictable, but determined and not easily influenced once my mind was set.

Things went well at West Haverstraw, and I believed that as time went by I would continue to improve physically. I had hope for the future as long as I remained where I was and kept receiving treatment. An added incentive was looking forward to the return of

Sue. Hopefully, her permanent presence would give me time to develop the kind of relationship with her that she expected. I was optimistic and felt good about things to come.

There was one concern, though. A high degree of muscle spasticity had developed in my lower back and legs, and this interfered with my everyday activities. Various treatments such as ice packs and muscle stretching were tried, but with little success.

Finally, it was suggested that I undergo a procedure known as a "phenol nerve block" in an attempt to reduce the muscle spasticity. The nerve block was to be a temporary condition lasting a maximum of six months, although its effect was said to have an unpredictable life span up to that time. Ideally, the nerve block would nullify all neural activity in those areas affected by the bothersome muscle spasticity.

The reasoning behind the nerve block was that if the muscle spasticity could be reduced, temporarily at least if not permanently, then I could continue to make progress in my physical therapy sessions that were now being hampered by the high level of spasticity. A go ahead stance already having been taken by both the ward doctor and my primary physical therapist, I was told to think over the matter and come up with my own decision.

Although I was aware of the problems caused by the muscle spasticity and didn't want it to stand in the way of my progress in therapy, still I wanted to speak with some of the patients who had undergone the nerve block and also with other hospital personnel who might have information about the procedure. With this in mind, I set out on my own pre-decision investigation.

The responses from patients who had experienced the phenol nerve block were largely negative. The results, I was told, were highly unreliable. In one case the desired effect lasted only a few hours. In another, the nerve block took away feeling that had been present before the procedure. Still another patient claimed that his ability to move one leg was lost following a phenol block. A final problem revealed to me was muscle contracture in the legs of a readmitted patient who had left the hospital after having the nerve block.

I next had a discussion with a male nurse who worked on our ward and seemed quite knowledgeable about the procedure. He told me that if phenol, or "carbolic acid" as it is known in its solution form, was injected into the vicinity of specific nerves it would have a nullifying effect on the nerves for an unpredictable period of time up to a maximum of six months. However, if the phenol happened to be injected directly into a nerve it would break down the nerve and destroy it. Hearing this certainly did no good as far as a pro vote for the nerve block was concerned. The nurse also said there was a similar procedure known as an "alcohol wash," which simply involved the use of alcohol rather than carbolic acid, that was entirely safe. This, though, was not even mentioned by either the doctor or therapists in favor of the phenol block.

My inner feeling was that I was at a crucial time during which I should let things progress naturally without chancing anything that might possibly interfere. Maybe the muscle spasticity would in time decrease, but even if it didn't I believed I could put it to work for me and actually use it to my advantage. For instance, leg bending and extension usually could be triggered by certain upper body movements. Also, the spasticity was maintaining good muscle tone in my legs; inactive muscles can soon lead to atrophy and contracture.

Although the level of muscle spasticity did pose some unwanted problems, I was not in favor of the phenol nerve block and therefore decided against it. I didn't realize, though, that being asked to think it over and come to a decision about the nerve block would take on two different meanings. To me it meant carefully weighing the pros and cons of the procedure given the evidence and information available to me, whereas to the ward physician it apparently meant having me decide just how soon I would be willing to go ahead with it.

I assumed that since I was given the option of making my own decision, a simple yes or no would be accepted and things would then continue on from there. Wrong assumption. Upon informing the ward doctor that I didn't feel the phenol nerve block would be the best thing for me I received the immediate and emphatic reply, "We'll decide what's best for you!" It was now clear that rejecting the nerve block risked discharge from the hospital. Besides staff belief that the degree of muscle spasticity present would hinder further rehabilitation progress, it also would not set a good example if a patient went against the recommendations and decisions of hospital personnel. This might encourage other patients to do the same, and that would pose problems for hospital policy. My feeling was that ultimately I had to answer to myself. What was best for me was what I myself decided. I didn't automatically and without question accept others' decisions about what I felt were important matters in my life, regardless of who those persons were or how right they thought they were. The final decision was mine. I owed that to myself; it is one of the responsibilities of living. Although I couldn't be absolutely certain, I believed I was making the right decision given the evidence and information available to me.

Following my rejection of the nerve block, it was concluded that I could no longer continue to make favorable progress with the degree of muscle spasticity present and therefore could not benefit further from remaining at the hospital, since I did not have any other medical problems requiring hospitalization. Arrangements for my discharge were made, a family conference was held, and I left the hospital in late November, four and a half months after having been admitted.

The original plan was for my rehabilitation to extend into the coming year by the time of its completion. An insurance company representative had told me my stay at the hospital would continue until around Easter. Declining the nerve block meant cutting my projected rehabilitation time in half. However, it basically came down to deciding between possible physical risks in terms of jeopardizing natural physical improvement, and an early end to my rehabilitation schedule. One decision or the other had to be made and I made the one I felt would be better in the long run, hoping I was right. My only concern now was my readiness to leave and reenter life in the outside world.

XIV. What Now?

Yesterday, all my troubles seemed so far away,
Now it looks as though they're here to stay,
Oh, I believe in yesterday.

Lyrics from "Yesterday"
The Beatles

During my stay at West Haverstraw I developed a dependency on and attachment to the hospital and people who worked with and assisted me in my daily living, many of whom I had come to know quite well. I felt as if I was a part of and belonged in the hospital, being equal to the other patients there and in harmony with and accepted by them. It was something I had gotten used to and with which I was comfortable.

I had fears about going back into the outside world again. My role in the hospital was easily defined and I had a clear and established identity there. I questioned whether I could function okay in the "real world" where everyone else did not have the physical limitations I did. Would I be able to fit in? Could I in this different world accept myself for what I was now, compared to what I used to be? It was going to be true test of readjustment, and not a simple one at that.

Being in the outside world again was scary and filled me with doubts and anxiety. This domain that before I so totally controlled now had me completely at its mercy. I was out of place and I knew it; I didn't fit in anymore. This world was for those who did things with physical ease and confidence, and that was no longer me.

My parents having divorced when I was young, I did not develop into a dependent family child and became somewhat aloof and self-reliant in my own unique and introverted way. At different times up through high school I lived with both my father and mother, then left to live in Cambria, Niagara Falls and Buffalo during my first years in college.

I had just returned to Western New York State from Indiana, where I was working and trying to finish college, when my accident happened. So, it was not surprising for me to be hesitant to give up the security I had during my stay at West Haverstraw. I didn't want to be dependent on my family the way I would once I left the hospital. I didn't know how to be and didn't know if I really could deal with that.

I knew I would have to leave the hospital someday, but wondered if I was truly ready now. I couldn't help having doubts about physically and psychologically making it. My mother had prepared for my arrival home, yet I wasn't sure I belonged there. But, my options were limited and I had no realistic alternatives. Home I would go, ready or not.

Returning home was a drastic letdown for me. It was like defeat. I had failed in my mission to overcome my injury. I had fought so hard to go to West Haverstraw because I felt it gave me the best chance for success. Now I was returning home before reaching the goals I had set. I was looking down a dead-end street once again and didn't see much ahead of me. Things didn't look good, and a growing low feeling began to set in due to my frustration and sense of futility.

Sue and I resumed our relationship upon my return home, but it soon became similar to the way it had been with Joyce. I placed the burden of keeping our relationship going entirely on Sue and was too unconcerned about it. Besides not putting enough into the relationship and giving the same effort as Sue, my not so good frame of mind caused laxness and uncertainty. Instead of contributing to our relationship, I was using all available energy within me to try to come to terms with myself. Sue sensed that my commitment was beginning to waver, and communication between us began to break down due to my lack of responsiveness and openness.

Coming home too soon was making it hard to adjust, and though I had related to Sue okay while in the hospital I wasn't able to do the same at home. It was clear that leaving the security of the hospital before I was ready was a liability to our relationship. Although we were now closer to one another in geographic distance, we were pursuing two different goals. What Sue wanted was to be loved and needed and to feel she was important to me. My foremost goal was to come to terms with my post-injury self, and until I could resolve everything inside me and adjust in some way to this new identity I wasn't going to be able to successfully have a genuine relationship with Sue, Joyce, or anyone else.

I just didn't have enough confidence in the future to give the energy and commitment needed to keep a relationship going. I was having a hard enough time trying to accept and relate to myself, so how was I going to accept and relate to someone else? In a true relationship the needs and interests of the other person are strongly in the forefront. My primary focus, though, was on myself and the uncertainty facing me. Unless I could come to terms and somehow function with my new identity, relations with both myself and others would not be easy. I had major problems, and only time was going to let me to work them out. If I could do that, I would be all right. I just needed some optimism and understanding about both myself and my future.

My main concern still remained, what was going to become of me and how was I going to deal with and overcome the restricting physical limitations with which I was saddled? Maybe there wasn't any way out, but only bad times and failure ahead. These were the concerns with which I had to deal, and finding acceptable solutions didn't seem easy.

Realizing our relationship was in trouble, by Christmas Sue and I let it come to a quiet and uneventful end without much fanfare. It just abruptly stopped without explanations or finger pointing and that was it. Sue recognized that I wasn't making use of her in the way she wanted. She expected to be a resource to me in my readjustment instead of having me shut her out and try to deal with things on my own. She had been right there for me to reach out to if that's what I was willing to do, just as earlier Joyce had been also.

My relationship failures with both Sue and Joyce showed the extent to which I had let my injury strip me of my sense of certainty, self-worth and control and, more importantly, my ability to closely and genuinely bond with another person in a mutually fulfilling way. In my fierce struggle to come to terms with my post-injury self I realized neither Sue, Joyce, nor anyone else could resolve my inner conflicts for me. That was something I would have to do on my own. It was selfish, inconsiderate and unfair to not have returned the same effort as Sue and Joyce in my relationships with them. Both had given genuinely of themselves in their relationships with me, and because my bond with her had developed deeper over a longer period of time it was Joyce in particular who deserved better than I was able to give. Yet I had nothing to be proud of in my relationships with either, and considering their sacrifices and efforts it was an injustice to them that I did not have the capacity to equally give back.

Having rejected the willingness of both Joyce and Sue to be a central and supporting part of my life, regardless of the uncertain turn it had taken, I was now left on my own to face whatever lay before me. It was time to seriously start looking at myself and my life situation, and come to some acceptance and understanding of them. Along with this, I wanted to see if something other than orthodox medicine could improve my physical condition.

After leaving the rehab hospital at West Haverstraw, I could see that medical technology as it then was could not reverse the physical consequences of spinal cord injury. When medicine fails people look elsewhere for answers, and I was no exception. One thing I looked at was charismatic religion, because healing was a big part of it.

It was Joyce who drew my interest to charismatic religion. Despite having turned away from her and gotten involved with Sue, being the special person she was Joyce did not let that break our ties to one another. Instead, once again she reminded me of her dedication and willingness to still be to me whatever I wanted her to be. As 1970 rolled around we began interacting some again, but although it was clear that Joyce had a degree of dedication that was rare to find, I still had not stabilized enough in my post-injury adjustment to accept her as a central part in rebuilding my life. Joyce was a religious person, and had hopes that I might be physically healed through the power of the Holy Spirit. One thing Joyce did was bring my attention to the healing ministry of Pittsburgh evangelist Kathryn Kuhlman. Kathryn Kuhlman was well- and widely known for her healing services. I traveled to Pittsburgh to attend one of these, but upon getting there the main part of the church where the service was being held was already filled so I ended up in the basement listening to the service over a speaker system. Not long after this Kathryn Kuhlman came to Buffalo, where a service was held in the large Kleinhan's Music Hall. Joyce wanted to go there with me, and we did get into the main part of the service. People came from everywhere to attend Kathryn Kuhlman's healing services held throughout the country, and the best advice was to arrive and line up early to stand a chance of getting into a service.

Persons were physically healed of major ailments at services conducted by Kathryn Kuhlman as agent of the Holy Spirit. There was no certainty, though, that attending a service would result in being healed. The amount of physical and emotional energy Kathryn Kuhlman put into her calling eventually became too great, and before long she took ill and died.

After the passing of Kathryn Kuhlman I attended other healing services, such as those of Fr. Ralph DiOrio of Leicester, Massachusetts, but again services of this type held no guarantees. What I learned about all of these services was that they should be attended for their value as spiritually fulfilling religious experiences and not with high expectation that healing would take place. Having continued expectations that go unfulfilled can cause great emotional stress and therefore be harmful to a person's sense of well-being. The main thing to realize is that, while healing is of great importance to anyone who truly needs it, the healing manifestations themselves are only an instrument of a higher purpose. The real purpose of healing services is the affirmation of religious faith and belief.

Joyce also was part of a small charismatic group whose leader was "Rev. Fred." Rev. Fred seemed to be a channel through which a power much greater than himself flowed, and he appeared to have genuine access to energy transmitted through his hands. This was evident when he stopped at our home one evening on his way to Rochester, saying that as he approached our house he was compelled by the Holy Spirit to stop. My aunt had driven out from nearby Lockport to visit me, and when my mother brought Rev. Fred into the kitchen where we were he asked if he could pray for and lay hands on me. When I said okay he really got into it and before long started speaking in tongues during the prayer. He was touching the top of my head and then slid his hands down to the location of my neck injury. Right at that instant that area of my neck began to vibrate strongly, but then Rev. Fred moved his hands away from that spot and the vibration stopped.

I didn't interrupt him to say anything because he was so much into the Holy Spirit that I didn't want to interfere with that, but I wonder what would have happened had I told him to put his hands back to where they had been. There definitely was some type of energy flowing from his hands, and maybe the very strong vibration I was feeling could have somehow affected in a healing way the nerve cells in my spinal cord had it continued. There's no way of knowing that now, though. It was, however, a very real physical experience. Rev. Fred moved to Rochester shortly thereafter, ending the opportunity for continued help in cultivating my spiritual awareness and acceptance, which were the keys to healing of both body and soul. God through Rev. Fred was ready to bestow whatever gift he had chosen, but I hadn't yet gotten where I needed to be in accepting it. I needed to put less emphasis on solely a physical healing for its own sake and more on true spiritual growth in the grander scheme of my existence.

I am a religious person who believes in the divine origin of the world and God's presence and influence in it. Yet, I realize that on earth we are physical beings bound by its physical laws and occurrences. Although there is help and guidance from Above when needed, there is not meant to be divine intervention at each and every step we make. That would take away the control and freedom of choice we were given and were meant to have in order to earn by our own decisions the worthiness on which we will eventually be judged. The spiritual realm is real and should be acknowledged and taken seriously because through our faith and actions we can be heirs to it, but it also has to be recognized that as human beings we are inescapably tied to the physical conditions and events with which we are faced while here on earth.

Sister Mary, from the hospital in Buffalo before I left for West Haverstraw in '69, made an important point. Serving as representative of my insurance company, she stopped by to see me during the summer after I had been at the rehab hospital at West Haverstraw. We talked about different things and the subject of faith healing came up. Sister commented, "You need to have faith in God, but you need to have faith in yourself also." What she was saying was that although you never give up your faith in and reliance on God, you also can't sit passively by waiting for things to be done for you. You have to take control to the extent you can, and achieve what you're capable of achieving with the inner resources you have and choices you make. In doing this, God will be there when you need and call on Him.

I realized it was time to start taking charge of my life to get it moving forward again. My approach to post-injury adjustment would have to be an inner process of close self-examination. I had to look deep within myself and completely restructure everything. I was going to have to honestly and directly evaluate every thought and emotion, both positive and negative, and resolve things the best I could. I had to cleanse my inner being and come to terms with myself. I had to face my conflicts head-on and come out a winner, no matter what.

I had to develop a new identity, one that reconciled past and present and accepted the best it could what now was. This would take time and a lot of soul-searching and self-judging, but it had to be done. Until the truism "Know thyself" became a reality for me, reclaiming a positive and successful status in life could not be achieved.

The task before me would involve getting my mind off my superficial exterior self and onto the processes of my inner self, which really determined who I was. All inner turmoil and confused emotional feeling had to be brought forth, faced realistically, and expelled with solution before I could take on a new, integrated identity. All sorts of powerful, repressed feelings and experiences rose with overwhelming force from within and left me emotionally drained, but at the same time a foundation was laid for the necessary reconstruction of who I was.

Good and bad had to be sorted out and separated, casting off all that was negative while keeping everything that would be beneficial and needed for favorable readjustment. With this accomplished, I was ready to be more accepting of my situation and go on from there the best I could. My spirit was too free to ever truly accept my changed physical being, but adjustment so I could function okay was something I could and had to do.

A readjustment of my values was also needed. I came to recognize the transitory nature of physical qualities and placed a new importance on those special, lasting qualities that make each person a unique individual. Qualities that, although not outwardly seen, are not fleeting but carry on and cannot be destroyed. What a person is goes beyond physical boundaries. In the end the physical self, while important in its own right, is but a secondary aspect of the true self that develops from within. Persons are, basically, what they themselves and others see them as being, and this is something that comes from inside. From the Old Testament comes the saying, "For as he thinketh in his heart, so is he." (Proverbs 23:7)

With a shift away from a physical approach toward life to one more mentally focused, my activities after leaving the hospital followed accordingly. While I did continue with physical therapy at home to try to maintain progress, I decided that it would be both creative and therapeutic to write a biography about my life's transition.

As summer came I also got the chance to continue my education with a couple of psychology courses at the State University of New York at Buffalo. In the second half of '68 I had been working toward my bachelor of arts degree in psychology there, and on the day leading up to my accident had been trying to cram in some studying for an upcoming final exam in one of my classes. Because of what happened that night, I never got a chance to take the exam back then. Now, though, I enrolled in a course and the professor was the same one I had for the class I never finished in '68. He said I could still take the final exam and he would then give me a course grade, so that worked out well.

What finally started pulling everything together for me was my decision in the early part of '70 to start writing the journal about all I had been through since my accident. This was a good therapeutic project for me. It helped me come to terms with much of the internal chaos within me and bought me to a greater overall understanding of things. By the time I finished the journal, I had purged from within me much of the unresolved turmoil that had been causing so many problems. I was now ready to look at things from a new perspective, and ready to start thinking about where to go next with my life.

During 1969 my problems relating to Joyce were something with which I couldn't deal. Now, though, my thoughts began returning to her. I was starting all over after having the first 22 years of my life suddenly yanked right out from under me, and it had taken time to begin putting everything back together. But when this did start to happen, Joyce was right back in my mind once more.

Before my sudden and unexpected injury, the holiday season at the end of '68 had given us a chance to see more of one another. There was a natural comfort being with Joyce and I looked forward to our times together. I didn't know just where our relationship was going in the upcoming year, but did know I wanted her to continue being part of my life. Would I have been ready to give the commitment then that I hadn't before completely given? I had the stability of a good job with a company that was paying for the remaining courses needed to complete my undergraduate degree and would pay for graduate degree courses after that. It didn't make sense continuing the noncommittal, freewheeling type of lifestyle I had been leading.

The year of '68 had been a time of opportunity, yet because of my hesitancy and excuses our relationship did not keep moving forward the way it would have had I been more dedicated to my role in it. The year ahead had the potential to be much more, but if it was it would be up to me to make it so. Joyce had already done all she could do. That's where we left off when I had the accident. It disrupted everything, and from that point I couldn't look at our relationship with any clarity until 1970 when I decided to talk with Joyce about what might still lay ahead in our lives despite all that had happened. I was ready to get my life going again, but no longer wanted to do it alone.

Being with Joyce the way I was now wasn't how I would have ever pictured or even wanted it to be, and I struggled as I wondered if the thoughts I was having were genuine and realistic. Were my reasons for thinking about having Joyce back in my life truly in her best interests or influenced more by the new life I now faced? And, could she really accept a future together with the dramatic change there had been, despite saying it hadn't made a difference? It would be much different than before, and there would be challenges. I wasn't sure how a talk between us might turn out, but I had to somehow get inside her mind, probe her feelings and find out before I could further move forward in restructuring my life.

The talk ended before it began. I heard that Joyce had gotten engaged and immediately dropped all thoughts of discussing anything with her. If she had the chance to have a happy and fulfilling life with someone who didn't have the physical limitations I did, then that's what I wanted for her. The best thing I could do now was just go on about my own business and not interfere.

It was ironic that the guy to whom Joyce had gotten engaged was the very person I had encouraged her to date while I was at West Haverstraw in '69. She had told me then that he kept asking her to go out with him, and she eventually did after I discouraged our relationship and became involved with Sue.

Although Joyce seemed uncertain, as if seeking answers as to just where her life too was headed at this time—answers I couldn't truthfully help her with now—she did get married in the fall of '70. She asked me to come to the wedding, but I knew I wouldn't. Without choice or resolution the bond between us had unwantedly been shackled by a reality that could not be changed, and the realization of that would have only magnified my discomfort in being there. My transformed physical status had taken away my options. I no longer was able to build our relationship into whatever I wanted it to be as I could have more easily done before. Had my accident not happened, at least I'd have had the chance to decide just what I wanted my future with her to be. Now, though, I felt I had no control over it at all.

This was something, though, on which I could not dwell. I certainly wished Joyce well, because she deserved whatever she could get out of life. But with or without her, what I needed to do now was get on with the task of rebuilding my life. If I had to go it alone at this point then that's what I'd do, but I needed to maintain a forward outlook.

I needed to put all of the past behind me. My pre-injury judgment and maturity had been far from being ideal. I wanted to start anew, a little older and hopefully much more aware of what relationships and life itself actually involved. It was time to admit the errors of my past and move on.

As fall marched forward I decided I did not want be to held hostage to the harsh weather all winter as I had the previous season. It was a disadvantage not being able to get out regularly and what I really needed, I felt, was to be in a milder climate. In a national spinal cord injury magazine I saw an advertisement about a residential medical facility for spinal cord injured persons in Guadalajara, Mexico. It was run and directed by an American physician and supposedly included therapy and rehabilitative services. I took an interest in this, contacted the physician, and made arrangements to go to Guadalajara. I figured that between the weather and the therapy

I might receive, I could make further progress in my rehabilitation. My aunt and brother-in-law flew with me from Buffalo to help me get set up in Mexico. We had a short layover in Dallas before continuing on to Guadalajara, and as we emerged from the plane there and were embraced by a surrounding blanket of 80-degree warmth I knew I wasn't going to have any complaints about the weather in Guadalajara.

We arrived at Guadalajara airport in the late afternoon and took a taxi to the medical facility. The weather, as expected, was sunny and fabulous. The doctor who was supposed to be there, though, was nowhere to be found. My residence turned out to be a small cottage and I didn't see any rehabilitation facilities. After talking to some of the workers, who didn't seem to know a whole lot about the situation other than that I was supposed to be assigned cottage space when I arrived, I started to get the feeling this place wasn't going to meet my needs and expectations.

I wasn't looking for a glorified nursing home that was a dead-end street. If there wasn't going to be a therapy and rehabilitation program, with a physician and therapists there to direct it, I wasn't interested and wasn't going to stay. I didn't want to just sit around and vegetate; I could do that anywhere. Granted the climate itself was almost enough to make me stay, but not quite enough.

The flight back to Buffalo wasn't until the next day, so my aunt and brother-in-law left to stay at the Guadalajara Holiday Inn while I spent the night in the cottage to which I had been assigned. I had an attendant who seemed a nice enough guy, but even the next morning there still was no sign of the physician.

My brother-in-law and aunt thought I should stay and give it a try, but my gut feeling was this wasn't the situation I thought it would be and as was presented. I had stayed awake all night thinking about it and by morning decided to leave. I wasn't about to take a chance this time and come out a loser. If I was going to leave, it had to be now.

We really had to do some finagling to arrange room for me on the return flight to Buffalo, but I was satisfied I had made the right decision in leaving and never had any regrets about doing so. I would just have to look at other options and try again.

The year of '70 had not been a good year. Rather, it was a continuation of all that had gone wrong since my accident. Within a span of less than two years, at a time when I should have had so much to which to look forward, I had lost two very important things in my life—the perfect health of youth and someone who had become much more a part of me than I had realized. There was usefulness after all in Sister's "face reality" approach to life. I had been living in a world of illusion. I believed nothing could stop me in life, but my injury very quickly shattered that illusion. And at the very same time, a relationship I thought would continue in the way I wanted came to an end in one moment in the darkness of a cold winter night. I hadn't been at all realistic.

It was completely back to the beginning to start over. In my life I had backtracked to the very bottom, and it looked as if the only positive thing left was there was nowhere to go but up. It was time to find out just what lessons I had learned, and this time see what I was really made of.

The arrival of 1971 seemed to hold potential for better things ahead. During the winter my dad by my mother's remarriage had spent much time converting a large commercial van into a motor home and as spring approached was anxious to try it out on a trip south to the sunny warmth of Orlando where my grandparents lived. Also on this trip were my mother, two of my younger brothers and myself. While in Orlando the man across from my grandparents' home took a strong liking to the motor home and before long its sale was being negotiated. He was originally from downstate New York, and since he wanted to return to New York State his Florida home across the street became part of the package. A deal was struck and there now was a house for our use when in Florida.

XV. Return to West Haverstraw

It was the summer of '71, and having spent a year and a half at home I felt as if I was stagnating. I had made some progress and reached a few goals, but still wasn't content with the way things were. What I needed, I believed, was a broader opportunity to make more happen in my life.

It was past time for a physical checkup, so I wrote a letter to the doctor under whose supervision I had been at West Haverstraw asking about being readmitted to the hospital for a follow-up examination and reevaluation. This was about the beginning of July, and just after sending off this letter I left with family for Orlando for two weeks. The house there bought earlier in the year was now vacant and available for use.

The time spent in Florida was a refreshing change. Also refreshing was an admittance notification from the rehab hospital awaiting me upon return to the North, although the speed of its arrival caught me off guard. I was to show up at the hospital that coming Monday. It already was the weekend, so I had to make fast arrangements.

I did arrive at the hospital on Monday, but not before the afternoon shift had come on duty. Most of the ward staff were well known to me from my previous stay at the hospital, which along with the familiar setting almost made it seem as if I had never left.

Aside from some different patients and a few new personnel, there was a comfortable familiarity to my return to West Haverstraw. One difference, though, was that before I had been on Ward A&B at the east end of the hospital. This time the hospital was in the midst of transferring A&B patients to Ward E&F, so for this stay I would be at the opposite west end of the hospital.

111

I at first thought I likely wouldn't be at the hospital much longer than it would take for a routine checkup and evaluation. Before long, however, I was approached with a proposal to participate in a study of an experimental drug that was thought to be effective in suppressing muscle spasms.

Since muscle spasms had been and still were somewhat of a nuisance to me I agreed to participate in the study, which was to continue for 15 weeks. During this time I was to be put on physical and occupational therapy programs and receive periodic evaluations in each. I also would be given a driving evaluation and have the opportunity to enroll in a couple of nighttime college courses that would begin at the hospital in September. All of this sounded good to me, and I was satisfied with my decision to stay and take part in the study.

One of the first persons I thought about from my previous days at West Haverstraw was a nurse's aide, Sally, who had worked the day shift on Ward A&B back then. Now on Ward E&F, I soon saw Norman, a male assistant who had also worked the day shift on Ward A&B in '69 but was assigned to Ward E&F's afternoon shift this time. While talking to him Norman asked, "Have you seen your girlfriend?"

I thought he was talking about Sue, and I told him that relationship ended shortly after I left West Haverstraw in '69. Norman said, "No, not that one…Sally!"

Sally wasn't my girlfriend. She was married for one thing, and back then the role of "girlfriend" was already filled by the complicated situation with Joyce and Sue. But Sally had been my favorite nurse's aide, and I enjoyed and looked forward to time spent with her on the ward. Norman's remark was simply his memory of the different way me and Sally interacted.

I was easygoing, not a demanding patient, and Sally was comfortable with me because I let her be however she felt like being around me. Sometimes we joked, sometimes we were serious, sometimes Sally had fun ribbing me, and sometimes she would be contently quiet in her thoughts without saying a word.

Sally usually was assigned everyday to help me with my morning routine on the ward, and this added something extra to each day. The freedom of shedding a rigid and expected role seemed to be important in Sally preferring to have me as one of her patients to assist. As with Sue when I had been hospitalized in Buffalo, the attention Sally gave me was something I looked forward to everyday and, because of that as well as the ease I felt and enjoyment I got from time spent with her, Sally was someone I truly missed after leaving West Haverstraw at the end of my first stay.

In attractiveness, Sally stood out among the other female staff on the ward and was a pleasant sight to wake up to each day. It was uplifting hearing her voice and laugh at the nurses' station when she arrived for work. I could always tell it was Sally coming down the ward aisle by the distinctive rhythmic "swish, swish, swish" sound her snug-fitting white button-down uniform dress made as she strutted along.

I missed Sally on her days off and always looked forward to her return. Her self-assurance, sassiness, fun and humor perked up the ward. But mostly I just felt more free and comfortable with her than with the other assistants, and enjoyed the interactions we had.

At West Haverstraw in '69 Sally was aware of my involvement with Sue, and had her fun with that. Sally and another nurse's aide, red-haired Beverly who usually was assigned to the opposite wing of the ward, were at the Spring Valley nightclub the evening Sue and I stayed at the Holiday Inn together. On Monday morning following that weekend, Beverly popped into my cubicle while Sally was with me and the two of them laughed and made insinuations as to what might have gone on between me and Sue at the hotel. I let them have their fun and didn't say anything, because what they were joking about hadn't happened. Sorry girls!

If there were going to be assumptions, Sue might have just as easily made her own. She arrived on the ward one morning when Sally and I were behind the drawn curtain of my cubicle. There was something amusing that we were both chuckling about, and Sue suddenly stuck her head through the curtain and questioned, "What's going on in here?!" Nothing—just the usual antics of me and Sally.

Now I was back at West Haverstraw two years later, wondering about Sally. Responding to Norman's question as to whether I had yet seen Sally, I told him I hadn't. Norman then emphatically advised me, "Then you'd better get down to Urology and see her, because that's where she is!" Sally had transferred to the Urology Department after my first stay at West Haverstraw.

The following day I showed up at the Urology Department. Sally was there, and it was good seeing her again. Yet, our interaction would be much different during this stay. Almost two years had passed since time together on Ward A&B in '69. That was a period of a relationship unique to then and there, and now was a different time and situation. But if I could have taken one person with me when I left in '69 it would have been Sally, because back then it was harder saying good-bye to her than anyone else as I left the ward and went out the door, leaving behind the security and daily reassurance of the hospital for the unknown world outside.

On Ward E&F, at first I was stuck in a small and cramped cubicle right next to the nurses' station, but soon there was a vacancy three cubicles down from where I was and I managed to shanghai this more spacious domain. Later still, I achieved the ultimate triumph by maneuvering my way into the sixth and last cubicle on the south side of the ward's west wing. Head day shift nurse, Pat, told me not to expect too much attention "way back there," but knew that was exactly what I wanted. Hidden away in the back corner of the ward was like being off in my own little world, and it gave me a unique sense of freedom and isolation. As a finishing touch I added a portable stereo phonograph I had recently purchased, for which I picked up new record albums during trips to huge Nanuet Mall a few miles south of West Haverstraw.

Things were easier and more enjoyable for me at the rehab center this time. I was stronger and more independent, and my attitude and state of mind were much better. Things meant more to me now, because my capabilities were greater and I was ready to use them to benefit both myself and others. Of special meaning was being able to lend a helping hand to those patients who were not at the stage I had reached. In turn, patients who were more able than myself did a lot to help me whenever I needed assistance with something I couldn't quite manage on my own. There existed a special sense of togetherness and common cause among the patients throughout the ward and hospital itself.

During this stay I saw once again some of the patients I had known during my first stay, since like myself other patients too were readmitted periodically for checkups or further treatment. Sadly, this was when I learned that 16-year-old Joey, who was fighting his drug dependence problem in '69, was now deceased from a self-administered drug overdose.

The summer of '71 was when the inmate riot at the New York State prison at Attica took place. There was a patient on my wing of Ward E&F, John, who had been an inmate at Attica. Officially, he still was an Attica inmate but had been sent to the hospital at West Haverstraw because of a spinal tumor he had developed. John had also been at West Haverstraw when I was there in '69, but on the opposite wing from me on Ward A&B.

John had been involved in a bank robbery, and using a shotgun had killed a security guard who was in pursuit. John was sent to Attica and while there developed the tumor that affected mainly his upper body function. With assistance he seemed to be able to stand okay.

During the Attica riot I sometimes stopped by John's cubicle and listened to radio news updates with him. He followed the unfolding of events closely throughout this time. John explained to me his role in the bank robbery and told about how the tumor had suddenly showed up.

I could sit and talk with John, yet it bothered me that he had deliberately killed another human being in the manner he did. John said it was either he or the guard, but I really had concern about someone robbing a bank with a loaded shotgun in the first place. Maybe the tumor was his karma. I hadn't ever robbed a bank or killed anyone, but looking back through my past I suppose I could have built up enough karma to have had my car tossed off the road and flipped. John may have developed the tumor, but he still had it comparatively good by being at West Haverstraw rather than Attica.

At the time of my return to West Haverstraw, Joyce and her husband Mike were living in Stony Point just a couple of miles north of the rehab center on Route 9W. After arriving at the hospital I learned they were making visits to a young girl on Ward A&B, and it was through Joyce and Mike that I met Laurie. Laurie was an exceptionally pretty girl about 10 years old with blazing red hair and freckles who was from an area of Western New York State near Rochester.

Tragically, Laurie had been struck by a truck near her home and sustained a high-level cervical spinal cord injury. She was totally paralyzed from the shoulders down and her breathing had to be assisted much of the time by a mechanical device. It was tough seeing someone so young in that condition, and it didn't seem at all right or fair.

Everyone liked Laurie, and her magnetic draw soon had me good friends with her too. I don't know how she managed to keep the sense of humor she so often showed, but I do know she was a very special and precious person. My heart went out to her parents, who clearly were themselves heartbroken to see their lovely, cherished daughter lying helplessly before them. I couldn't begin to imagine the pain, aguish and heartache they had to have been experiencing. It was a heartrending nightmare, nothing less, and something almost too cruel to accept.

Rejecting the harsh reality before me, I would gaze at Laurie while my mind drifted to images of her running free and unfettered, her long shining hair flowing majestically behind her in the wind. That's the way Laurie was meant to be. What kind of a world was this in which something so devastating could happen to someone so innocent and deserving? My injury and why it occurred was understandable and I could deal with it because of that, but the helpless pain I felt for Laurie was something very different.

Since Laurie seemed to take a special liking to me, I would often stop by her ward to see her. Then as the staff began trying to gradually wean her from assisted breathing, sometimes her parents or someone from her ward would bring her to my ward for a visit. On her ward Laurie had use of a more elaborate breathing assist device. Off the ward, to provide extra oxygen when needed, it was usually enough for someone to squeeze air into Laurie's lungs using a manual hand bag apparatus.

Knowing I would soon be starting my two evening college courses at the hospital, American Literature and Psychology of Adjustment—a fitting course for sure to be offered at the rehab center—Laurie gave me a composition notebook. On the inside cover of the notebook was written, "To Ron. Love Laurie." It was a very special gift from a very special person and something to treasure because of that.

The daytime head nurse on Laurie's ward was in my Psychology of Adjustment class. When the class first began the instructor asked each person how much psychology instruction he or she previously had. By this time I had taken plenty of psychology courses, including child psychology, and when I told the instructor how many hours of psychology background I had Laurie's ward nurse said to me, "Wow, no wonder you're so good with Laurie!"

But, it wasn't psychology I used with Laurie. I was just genuinely relating to her as one person who cared about another, that was all, and that was good enough for Laurie.

Spinal cord injury is not a good thing to have happen at any age. At least I had gotten the chance to fully experience my younger times, making it through almost 23 years of life before meeting the misfortune I did. Laurie hadn't and, even worse, the degree of her injury was much more severe. Her high level of injury left her with virtually no movement and difficulty with her breathing. Tragically the breathing problem would eventually get the best of Laurie, even though she had the spirit of a fighter.

After Laurie left the hospital to return home, the worst that could happen did. She developed respiratory complications that she could not overcome. What happened to Laurie affected me, because if everything she went through could befall someone so angelic and innocent, then life surely had no fairness to it at all. It was hard to understand. What a loss to her parents and to everyone who knew her! It made me question a lot of things, but I didn't come up with any satisfactory or acceptable answers. But if ever there was a time for faith and hope for better things beyond the present world we know, this was surely it.

There was a gentleman on our ward somewhat older than the average patient, typically in the late teens or early twenties, who had gotten injured when he fell out of a tree while picking apples. He wasn't severely incapacitated and could walk okay with the assistance of two canes. His cubicle was directly across from mine, and at this time I was on a dressing program designed by my physical therapists, Louise and Kathy. That meant that each morning I had to put on by myself socks, undershorts, tee shirt, trousers, shirt and shoes. When I first started the program, dressing would always take quite a while, but Louise and Kathy insisted that I get it done each morning.

The toughest part was my trousers, and one morning I had gotten that far but was struggling a bit. The guy across from me had been watching with amusement and finally asked, "Need some help?"

"Sure," I said. I was anxious to finish dressing and get off the ward.

He came over and was helping me get the trousers in their final position when lo and behold Louise and Kathy came walking onto the ward. They spotted us and threw a fit. My accomplice scrambled out of there in a hurry, and after a stern lecture I was left to put back on the trousers Louise and Kathy removed so that I would have to start over. Louise smiled in a sort of "We gotcha!" way and said, "See you down at PT when you finish, Ron," which took a while.

Working on homemaking skills was part of my occupational therapy program. Before my injury I was quite used to homemaking tasks because of the time I had spent living by myself, and I really didn't mind them at all. It was tougher doing it now, although with effort I could still get the job done. To successfully complete the program I had to pass a final evaluation. Among the evaluation tasks were vacuuming a rug, making a bed, and preparing a meal.

I got the floor clean and got all the folds on the bed right. The meal actually was going to be the fun part, because I was allowed to choose what to prepare and also allowed to invite a guest. I invited a fellow "quad" and good friend from Ward E&F, Gary, who was from the Buffalo suburb of Tonawanda, very familiar territory from my pre-injury days.

The meal I choose was hamburgers and chef salad, accompanied by milk. I had to form hamburger patties, flip them as they cooked, and then serve them in hamburger rolls. This wasn't too hard. The salad was a bit trickier, because I had to slice tomatoes and cut up other vegetables. Once that was done, though, it was just a matter of adding salad dressing and the vegetables to broken up lettuce and mixing everything together. When it was all over, I had passed with rave reviews.

It was good to polish up on my homemaking skills because of my plans to go to Florida following my discharge from the hospital, even though when I left for Florida I most likely wouldn't be going there entirely on my own. But, I had made up my mind that after leaving the hospital I wasn't going to return to Western New York State and resume any kind of restricted lifestyle. With all due respect and gratitude for the help and steadfastness of my family, I knew my future was not in returning home this time but rather striking out in the world on my own. Florida would present a new environment and a new lifestyle. In a sense it would be like starting over in life and building from there.

On Ward E&F was a young bearded quadriplegic fellow, Bob, who one day came up with the idea of racing me around the entire main circular corridor of the hospital, starting at a begin/end point outside of the gift shop near Ward A&B. To the victor would go the proceeds of a $1 bet just to make the race more interesting.

Bob got off to a flying start and good lead, but then I caught up to and passed him. I got far enough ahead so that as the corridor turned just enough I was out of Bob's sight. Shortly beyond this point was an incline that took some effort to go up. Someone came walking up behind me and asked if I needed assistance going up the incline and I said sure, that would be appreciated. With this bit of help I was up the incline in no time and headed for the turn that would send me whizzing down the slope in the corridor heading for the halfway mark of the race.

I really made good time from that point on, and when I came full circle to the starting point by A&B I saw Bob coming back down the same stretch of corridor where he had at first gotten off to such a good start. Apparently he had trouble with the incline, which was fairly steep for someone not having strong arms, and turned around. Bob started to get out his dollar, but I told him to keep it. I didn't tell him I hadn't won entirely on my own, but at the same time didn't dare take the dollar for winning because my conscience wouldn't let me do that. I had such a good lead that I'm sure I would have won anyway. It's just that I wouldn't have made it completely around so fast without help going up the incline.

I was fast enough for the arm muscle limitations I had, but my little 14-year-old paraplegic friend from Ward E&F, Melvin, was someone who could really burn up the tires. He would start at one point, take off down the corridor on his two back wheels, and come flying around to the starting point in no time flat. Melvin and I remained buddy-buddy until another patient, Linda, and I started to hang around together. Then Melvin got upset because he liked Linda, even though she was five years older than he. In time, though, Melvin accepted the fact that he was just a bit too young for Linda and I wasn't.

When autumn came and the weather turned cooler, I liked the warmth that the cast-iron steam heat radiators gave off. I would position myself beneath them in the corridors and on the ward in an effort to stay warm, because I didn't like being cold. Often in bed on the ward it was like an all or nothing thing, though, because the radiators would give off heat to the point that the windows had to be opened to counteract it.

I participated in more recreational activities during this stay at the hospital. I went along on several outings and excursions and attended many on-grounds functions such as movies, musical performances, parties and cookouts. Also I would often go out on weekends when visitors came, as well as going out sometimes on weekday nights. Occasionally weekends provided the opportunity for visits home. As one weekend approached one of my physical therapists, Kathy, said she would be going right by Buffalo on a visit to family in Canada. Kathy offered to drop me off in Royalton Center where I had been staying with my mother and family. I accepted her offer and Kathy told me she would stop at the hospital for me early Saturday morning.

Saturday morning Kathy and her younger sister pulled up outside Ward E&F in Kathy's Plymouth Duster as scheduled. It looked as if they were already prepared for lunch. They had sacks of food and a bottle of Boone's wine. As we were driving along Kathy thought she could do better than the radio, so she turned it down and sang "Mercedes Benz," one of Janis Joplin's songs. Move over Janis; Kathy did all right.

When we left Royalton Center on our return trip to West Haverstraw, Kathy had driven a few miles to as far as a blink on the map along Route 77 called Basom when she looked in the rear view mirror and saw a brown Buick Electra coming up on us fast. Kathy remarked, "Hey Ron, I think your mother's behind us." Sure enough, we had left without a lunch package Mother had made up. At least she caught up to us before we had gotten completely out of the area. Come to think of it, at times she was a little heavy on the gas pedal.

As we were passing the shopping Center on Route 9W south of Haverstraw, Kathy noticed that the movie "Summer of '42" was playing. She wanted to come back later and see it, but I knew once I got back to the hospital I'd probably just settle in for the evening, and her sister didn't seem overly enthused. What a couple of stick-in-the-muds!

It was Kathy who tagged me with the nickname, "The Priest." I reported to the Physical Therapy Department one day for a mat exercise class conducted by Kathy and my other physical therapist, Louise. My lunch mate friend Gary, who was also in the mat class, had gotten hold of a stack of *Playboy* magazines that someone had brought into the PT Department and was passing around. Gary offered me a magazine but I said no thanks. I wasn't interested and wanted to get started with mat class. So, Kathy started assisting me in some mat work while Gary continued to focus his attention on the magazines.

Kathy labeled me The Priest for turning down the magazines. If I wanted to read it would be one of my American literature or psychology books, but my priority now was physical therapy and I was going to get in my full session of mat work. While at West Haverstraw for this stay, I was seriously and strongly focused on achieving as much as I could physically and didn't intend to miss even one minute of my scheduled therapy time.

Now that I had the new nickname, I decided to put it to use. In the corridor outside the Education Department I came upon Linda, the heartthrob of my little buddy Melvin who now was once again hanging around more and more with me, and she asked me to sign her leg cast. A bit to Linda's surprise and wonderment, on the cast I wrote a short notation and signed off as "The Priest."

During this stay at West Haverstraw I frequently got away from the hospital to do one thing or another. When professional football season started in the fall, the Recreation Department arranged trips to Yankee Stadium in the Bronx where the New York Giants played and I went to some of these games. It was quite pleasant sitting in the early autumn sunshine when the Giants played the Baltimore Colts and Pittsburgh Steelers during the first part of the season.

Later in the season, though, when the weather was much cooler and there was a biting frigid wind blowing through Yankee Stadium, I attended a Giants versus Minnesota Vikings game and just about froze. Julie, a physical therapist who had come along on the outing, wrapped me in a wool blanket like a mummy and hugged me to keep me warm. That should have done it because a good-looking girl like Julie shouldn't have had any trouble turning my blood warm and under normal circumstances probably wouldn't have. Nevertheless, I was still looking forward to some indoor shelter and hot coffee. I glanced up to see skittery Giants' quarterback Fran Tarkenton scrambling all over the field as usual, the weather not seeming to bother him at all.

Besides football games, other outings away from the rehab center included a nighttime tour of New York City with Alan, the head nurse on Ward E&F during the 3 to 11 P.M. shift, on one of his evenings off duty. During our tour in the little Volkswagen he was driving that night, Alan pointed out the different boroughs and we buzzed into Manhattan where the nighttime streets were surprisingly deserted. Like a mouse scurrying through a looming mansion, as it puttered along our tiny, toy-like scoot-about seemed dwarfed by the surrounding urban immensity engulfing it.

While zipping around Manhattan, Alan pulled up beside a building on a darkened side street and briefly went into an apartment of someone he knew. As I waited alone in the car until he returned I began wondering about the possibility of getting mugged. Being in New York City for the first time, I was intimidated by its unfamiliarity and the misconceptions about it in my mind. I kept glancing about nervously to distinguish figures emerging from the shadows and kept a keen ear for the sound of approaching footsteps. Since he knew it better, Alan had a lot more confidence in the city at night than I did and there didn't turn out to be any threats other than the ones in my imagination.

When a big state funding hearing for the hospital was held in New City just a few miles south of West Haverstraw, I attended it with Alan. He picked me up at the hospital in the morning and we drove to the City Hall in New City where the hearing was held.

The hearing was mostly an all-day affair, but we couldn't stay the entire time because I had one of my experimental drug evaluation sessions scheduled for that afternoon and had to return to the hospital. When I told Alan I had to be back at the hospital that afternoon he exclaimed, "What?!" He was looking forward to having lunch at a nice restaurant and having a leisurely day out. We ended up going to McDonald's in New City and then headed back to West Haverstraw. Alan seemed to take it in good stride, though.

When I reported for my evaluation session and said I had just returned from the hearing in New City, Kris, the lab technician who tested me regularly told me she wished I had said I would be going to the hearing. She wanted to go too and had only stayed at the hospital for my testing session. Kris said we could have canceled that day's session. Two disillusioned people in one day—I think I needed to sharpen up a bit on my interpersonal communication skills!

In October the Hudson Valley came alive with emblazoned foliage at the height of its colorful, chameleon-like change. Saturating the visual senses, a chromatic spectrum of indescribable wonder burst forth in its vivid presence, the awesome product of the incomparable touch of God's own creative hand.

Amidst this, the Education and Recreation departments jointly scheduled a Saturday trip to Bear Mountain State Park just north of the hospital between Palisades State Parkway and Route 9W. Many of the teachers at the hospital came along to escort the patients, and anyone who wished was given a camera and color film with which to take pictures. Music teacher, Rose, offered to accompany me. When I first met her during my '71 stay at the hospital she remarked, "Your reputation has preceded you," apparently referring to my previous stay in '69 before she started working there. I wasn't sure just what she had heard about me, but judging from the upbeat tone of her comment I assumed it was more positive than not.

Comparable in youthful freshness to the beauteous flower bearing her name and favorably competing with the splendor of nature's autumn marvel, Rose's presence was a pleasant bonus that added to my enjoyment of the outing. It was a stunningly gorgeous Indian summer day displaying a magnificent leaf and foliage palette—spectacular reds, yellows, oranges, browns and golds. As I basked in the bright, warm sunshine and watched, Rose artistically designed several colorful leaf collages and took pictures of them.

The only unpleasant thing during the trip happened after we had reached the top of Bear Mountain and were making our way back down along the side of the mountain's main access road. Being with Rose, I was doing all right going down the slope. One of the patients, however, teenage Randy from Ward G&H who generally was able to handle his chair okay by himself, suddenly ran into trouble with the steepness of the downward grade of the road.

Randy was at the hospital because of a head injury, and had arm and leg impairment on one side of his body. On level ground he was doing all right handling his chair, but then all of a sudden downhill momentum got the best of him.

Almost immediately at the edge of the road was a fairly steep drop-off, the redeeming factor being that at least it did fall straight down to nowhere. All I know is one moment Randy was there and the next moment he wasn't. For a stunned second or so everyone was frozen in time while what had just happened was being mentally processed. Then one of the male teachers frantically scrambled down the side of the drop-off and unbelievably somehow managed to reappear again carrying in his arms a very scared and shaking, but still alive, Randy.

Although miraculously not seriously injured, Randy was bruised and cut up enough so that he had to be immediately taken back to the hospital for treatment. He ended up with soreness and some stitches, but it could have been much worse. It was a shocking and seemingly unreal thing to have happen on an outing where everything was supposed to be fun and enjoyment.

The Education Department sponsored an evening trip to Tappan Zee Playhouse in nearby Nyack where the classic film "Citizen Kane" was showing. It was late fall so the weather was quite crisp. The film was fine, but afterward people wanted to stop at an ice cream parlor in Nyack. Me and my friend Gary didn't favor that, but reluctantly went along with the crowd.

By now Linda and I were spending more time together, so this outing was like a date for us. She and her rock 'n' roll fanatic friend Mary thought the ice cream parlor idea was great, as did most

125

everyone else. Our join-in participation would have put Gary and me at risk of becoming innocent victims of negligent homicide, because we were warmth people who weren't about to consume ice cream and cold drinks when it was almost ready to snow outside.

We would have been satisfied if we could have at least gotten some coffee, but there was none—no hot coffee, no hot tea, no hot chocolate, no hot anything! Questioning their sanity, as Gary and I glanced around everyone else seemed to be having a good ol' time. I was shivering too much to do a lot of talking, but I was doing plenty of thinking about my cozy cubicle back at the rehab center with the trusty steam radiator on the wall above it casting off toasty rays of comforting heat.

Going shopping at Nanuet Mall was something I liked to do, and I was able to get there fairly often. Nanuet Mall was a large, two-story mall with a flat conveyor belt escalator that made access between floors very easy. New clothes were favorite items purchased during my shopping trips, as were record albums. With my shopping excursions and all of my other various outings, I got time away from the hospital on many occasions.

As for my participation in the experimental drug program, once a week I would report to a research office located in the Physical Therapy Department for an afternoon testing session, the purpose of which was to determine the effects of the medication I was taking. The experiment was "double-blind," meaning that neither I nor the research assistant who did the weekly evaluations, the earlier-mentioned Kris whose attendance at the hospital funding hearing I had thwarted, knew for certain exactly when I was on or off the drug. In one phase of the experiment I would be taking the real thing, and in another, placebos or fakes.

The study was headed by one of the hospital's research doctors but most of my contact was with Kris, who wasn't much older than me. The usual testing session would begin with Kris checking my blood pressure and testing my neural reflexes. I would then be placed on my stomach on an examination table and electrodes would be inserted at nerve sites feeding various leg and foot muscles.

Electrical nerve impulse activity could then be recorded and also artificial stimulation of muscle activity initiated as desired. During one part of the experimental session I would remain passive, and during a second part I would be asked to try to initiate certain leg movements through my own conscious effort.

The results of these experimental sessions, together with regular interval blood and urine analysis and physical therapy testing evaluations, indicated how the drug program was progressing.

I didn't like the light-headedness or "high" that the medication sometimes produced, but some patients who were not on the drug heard about this effect and tried to get me to give them some of the large supply I was given as my discharge from the hospital approached. My answer was no. Not only did the mediation I was given have to last until I returned for reevaluation in a few months, but also I didn't feel it was right to hand out drugs for any other purpose than the original medical intention.

Those asking me for medication needed more than the superficial lift it might have given them. They could have filled any troubling void within them by going to the church services Sundays in the hospital's auditorium. That would have brought deeper meaning and been a truer answer to what they really were seeking.

For participating in the study I was entitled to a free supply of muscle spasm medication for as long as I wanted. I would continue to take the medication for a period of time following release from the hospital as part of the follow-up on the drug, but after my obligation of taking it was over I eventually discontinued it because, for one thing, I didn't like its side effects. Also, I didn't need to keep taking the medication on a continual basis since the degree of muscle spasticity had greatly diminished and was not that much of a problem anymore. The pharmaceutical company had already gotten the needed data from my participation in the research study, and that was the main thing.

Side affects of the medication for me included light-headedness, unexplainable skin conditions, and hair loss. There were reports of liver problems in some persons, but I never experienced that. The thing that bothered me most was the hair loss. Mornings I would wake up to find numerous strands of hair scattered on my pillow. Thin hair and a receding hairline were characteristics of older males on my father's side of the family, but I didn't want to start having hair loss even before I turned 30.

I was glad to have helped in the study, but for me the drug was something I felt should not be taken for an extended period of time, especially if there were going to be side effects. I believed drug free was the way to be unless I clearly had to take medication, which at that time I didn't.

XVI. A Marginal Man in a Marginal Land or...A World of No Return

He's a real nowhere man,
Sitting in his nowhere land,
Making all his nowhere plans for nobody.

Lyrics from "Nowhere Man"
The Beatles

Back at West Haverstraw in the summer of '71 I was at a point of crucial transition in my life. I still clung to the ideal image of my pre-injury life, yet knew that in reality my past and present were two dramatically different and irreconcilable worlds. But the past was good and held much promise, and I fought strongly against giving up the future potential it held.

Joyce was a vestige of the world I knew at the time of my accident, and still being in my presence she was a key symbol representing my struggle to differentiate the opportunities of that life from the uncertainties to be faced in this new life ahead of me. In returning to West Haverstraw I in no way intended to re-involve myself with her. She was now married and I considered our ties a clear and decided thing with a distinct separation between past and present.

Joyce's marriage was not working, however, and when I realized she wanted out of it I couldn't help thinking about what that meant in terms of my relationship with her. There had been much change in both of our lives since my accident, yet I still felt a lingering connection to her. Yet how could three unwanted years of what we had both experienced be erased and a life that existed before reclaimed? How could we go back after such disruption and change and continue on as if nothing had happened? I didn't want anything to do with my present life, but there it was. I preferred the past, though in reality it was gone and wasn't going to come back.

The idealistic images I held of both Joyce and myself no longer existed. Physically I had changed and my image of Joyce had changed because of her marriage to Mike. Yet her ongoing presence offered a chance to hold on to a part of the pre-injury life I had lost, so there was a reluctance to completely let go of that. Even though the physical consequences of my accident were the ultimate deciding factor in determining my relationship with Joyce from that point on, nonetheless she symbolized the pre-injury life to which I wanted to return. Her presence was a constant reminder of the unresolved marginal world in which I was now caught.

By early fall Joyce told me she was leaving Mike. As a couple, it was up to Joyce to decide how compatible she and Mike were. Whatever problems existed between them, from talking to her I could see she had made up her mind to end her marriage.

With images of the past crowding my mind, I felt the sharp sting of blame for the less than ideal situations in which we both now found ourselves. At the end of summer in '68 Joyce had asked for an enduring commitment. And she didn't necessarily expect an immediate walk down the aisle but rather simply an assurance that our relationship meant enough to me for it to be a lasting thing, no matter when it was formally made a permanent union. Because of what she had put into the relationship Joyce had every right to expect that from me and made her feelings known in good faith, relying on me to respond in a genuine and committed way. But I wasn't yet ready to settle down and didn't give that assurance. I was too caught up in the illusions of my free and fast-paced living to be able to look beyond it and see Joyce's more sane and realistic view of things.

Not only would the commitment Joyce wanted have met the expectations she had, but it also would have put me in a more responsible and lower risk pattern of living that might have saved both of us from going through all we had since my accident. I could have spared each of us unnecessary and difficult times by having been more settled and mature. That immaturity and unsettledness was a serious flaw that had affected both Joyce and me, and I was now staring directly at its destructive consequences. What had happened to me I had done to myself. It was Joyce who was the true victim and that was neither right nor fair. Negatively affecting my own life was one thing, but I didn't have the right to similarly affect someone else's life too, and perhaps I was now justly paying the price for that.

During the fall Joyce continued to come to the rehab center to see me and Laurie, and nights or on weekends she at times would free me from the hospital setting by taking me to places such as the Nanuet Mall where I liked to shop. At the hospital itself we did simple things such as strolling around or just visiting together.

One day we went for a walk to the picnic area across the service road from Ward E&F. We singled out a picnic table and began to talk. As we chatted the wind picked up and the sky darkened. Giving an upward glance at the ominous clouds fast closing in on us Joyce warned, "I think it's going to pour any second."

With a gaze skyward I nonchalantly replied, "It looks like it's a ways off yet." Right after saying that a downpour began and we got soaked to the skin by time we made it back inside. I should have listened to Joyce.

The caught-in-the-rain incident seemed to represent in a microcosm how the larger relationship between us had typically been. Whereas for Joyce it had always been a simple thing to sense just how and in what time frame our relationship was supposed to unfold, I had a harder time recognizing and accepting that. What was for sure, though, was that I could have benefited from listening more closely to Joyce and settling down before what eventually happened to me did.

After Joyce's breakup with Mike there continued to be much debate within me about what exactly my relationship with her was to

131

be. Although by this time I had met and begun to develop a relationship with Linda, I wondered if Joyce might still be the woman in my future. Past ties to her remained, but I was struggling with the effect that both my accident and Joyce's marriage had on my expectations for a true relationship with her.

It was difficult knowing just what was going on in Joyce's head, so it was a somewhat uncertain situation. Although she had intentionally made the move she did and was serious about ending her marriage, I couldn't clearly figure out whether or not she had hopes that I might still have an interest in her. Whatever interest I did have, the opportunity was now there to act on if I was going to.

Making herself vulnerable in the past, Joyce had been open and trusting but had not gotten from me the return response she should have. It seemed as if she was throwing out innuendos, though at the same time there appeared to be hesitation to once again take risks. Moreover, she was aware of the presence of Linda and it likely didn't take much imagination to envision parallels with the Sue escapade during my previous stay at West Haverstraw.

Yet despite the potential that existed with Linda, and it was a potential that was real, Linda was someone new to me so Joyce's importance carried is own weight because of our past ties. By leaving Mike Joyce had made resuming a relationship with her possible, but if that's what I wanted it would be up to me to communicate that to her. Joyce was no longer taking things for granted, and looking back through the history of our relationship that was quite understandable.

All along, my relationship dependability had never centered as much on my capacity to give a genuine and steadfast commitment as getting to the point where I was truly willing to do that. But, what good really was commitment willingness now? Still in the very forefront loomed the complicated and possibly insurmountable factor of my post-injury self-identity.

My ideal image of being with Joyce was one in which my injury had never occurred, because for me that was something that simply should not have happened. Joyce had made it clear to me earlier, however, that my accident had not changed her way of thinking about our relationship. So even though I did not respond to that at the time, as far as I was concerned that's the way things last stood. Until Joyce indicated that she had different feelings now, I was going to proceed on that premise. I was going to take everything into consideration and then come up with the best decision I could. And if I did decide to try again, I knew the only outside factor that could yet stand in the way would be reluctance on the part of Joyce herself.

Nonetheless, I still had some serious questions with which to struggle within myself. Aside from continuing serious concerns about whether or not a post-injury relationship with Joyce could really be, there remained one other very crucial hurdle to clear and that was the issue of her marital status.

During my decision dilemma I got a lot of unsolicited input from others who took notice of my interactions with Joyce. Head nurse Alan warned me not to get involved with a woman who was still legally married, because if I did I might find myself named a corespondent in a divorce suit. Saying he was speaking from personal experience, Alan felt he had grounds to advise me.

This point bothered Alan more than it did me, so I wasn't too concerned about it and didn't give it much serious thought. It was a legal issue that wasn't as important to me as just coming to a personal decision of whether or not I should go ahead with what I was debating in my mind about Joyce. We certainly weren't seriously involved in any way and weren't having any kind of physical affair, and therefore I wasn't concerned that I was involved in anything like adultery.

I wasn't trying to interfere with Joyce's marriage, and Joyce wasn't the type of person to intentionally put me in a difficult situation. Our relationship wasn't devious or a threat to anyone. I realized that right at this time Joyce and Mike were only separated, not divorced, so my involvement with her necessarily had to be limited. It was clear, however, that before long Joyce was going to be a free woman again, so all I wanted was to figure out if I should go ahead with plans regarding her on that basis. The fact was that, regardless of my presence, the relationship of Mike and Joyce as

the back injury. I thought only cats landed on their feet when they
fell.

George favored my relationship with Joyce, but in listening to
him comment about her physical attractiveness and the sporty car she
owned I knew I wasn't going to pay much attention to him. He was
interested in superficial and material things, and they weren't
foremost in my mind. Instead, I wanted to go beyond the surface and
get in touch with what lay much deeper.

My own thoughts about Joyce were focused on her overall
qualities as the person I had come to know and be connected to over
the years I had known her, with her true inner self and natural and
enduring ties to me being what mattered most. Joyce truly was an
exceptional person, and on impulse alone it would have been very
easy to go in her direction. My days of impulsiveness, though, were
over. The inescapable fact was that Joyce did not have something
very important to me, and that was the marital status of single, never
married.

Alan's warning against getting involved with a married woman
made me realize that Joyce's marital status was indeed a key issue,
not for the reason Alan had given but for my own very personal
reasons. No matter how I tried to see her as being, because she had
already married someone else Joyce just wasn't the same person to
me she had been before. My special image of her was what I had
known before her marriage. And very likely her true image of me was
my pre-injury image, minus, of course, the frustrating noncommitment
I had then displayed. So neither of us was to the other what we had

previously been, and that was something we could not go back and reclaim.

Life has a distinct time perspective. Things are real and possible as they are happening, but once their time has passed they are gone. To be solid and pure of bond, relationships in particular need an unbroken continuation. Once broken, the best that can be is to cherish a relationship as the positive and enriching experience it was. It is the meaning felt as memories fill the mind that gives to a relationship forever the fulfillment and specialness it had during its time.

My bond with Joyce and images of the past had fueled thoughts about her that could not be. When I stopped to think about it and faced the real truth, even though her marriage did matter, despite anything else the one unchangeable thing that steered the course of everything between us since the time of my accident was that at the moment my injury happened whatever future potential still ahead of us was lost.

Seeing before me the truth of my present life, my mind was now made up to not pursue things further with Joyce. She wasn't the answer to what I really had so desperately been seeking, which was the waving of a magical wand that would make disappear my spinal cord injury and all of its negative consequences. I was ready to accept a permanent partner in life, but now knew it was going to be someone I had met after my injury and not before it.

This final resolution of my long and uncertain relationship with Joyce was a key to giving up the idealism of the past and accepting the realism of the present and future. Having at last let go of a primary symbol still binding me to my pre-injury life, I could now go forward with all of the accomplishable possibilities of the future. I emerged from my marginal world of uncertainty and reluctance to give up the past, and was now ready to embrace as best I could a future before me with a realistic view of my true present self.

Regardless of how things turned out, I owed much to Joyce. She left me something very valuable, and that was the realization of just how important true genuineness and steadfastness are in human relationships. There was a feeling of melancholy in having to move on, because there weren't that many people like her out there in the world.

In my pre-injury life I was fortunate to have received God-given gifts and blessings, gifts and blessings that I failed to recognize, appreciate and thankfully embrace because I was too focused on myself and my misguided way of living. I did not look upward with acceptance and grateful acknowledgement to their true source. Gifts, when given, must be accepted and valued as they are meant to be or risk being lost. Self-focus and wrong life choices had resulted in the loss of much of the potential that the future held. I now found myself in a totally different world—my post-injury life—and I could not again make the mistake of not recognizing and accepting new gifts given.

XVII. Then Comes Marriage

Saying before returning to West Haverstraw that I needed a broader opportunity to make things happen in my life may have been an understatement. Without knowing exactly where everything was leading, events began to take their own course once I was back at the rehabilitation center. I simply became part of that situation at that time and place, and consequently became part of all that was then unfolding. The breakup of Joyce's marriage and my initial thoughts about her were one thing. Something else unfolding at West Haverstraw during this time was a growing relationship with a patient on Ward A&B.

I first saw 18-year-old Linda at West Haverstraw when she came to the hospital from her home in Brooklyn for an outpatient orthopedic clinic visit. My first awareness of her was more auditory than visual, since I was on my wing of Ward E&F when she came up to the nurses' station in the corridor outside the wing and began openly greeting people she knew from her previous stays at and clinic visits to the hospital. I glanced out into the corridor and saw a short, bubbly brunette who seemed to know very well all of the staff and many of the patients.

Linda had noticed me earlier in the main hospital corridor, and before leaving E&F asked her close friend Mary, a spina bifida patient on the opposite wing of the ward, who I was. Then Linda said with certainty to Mary, "He's the man I'm going to marry."

After her clinic evaluation, Linda was admitted to the hospital to have surgery on her foot. The surgery was needed because of Linda's congenital orthopedic condition, medically known as "arthrogryposis," resulting from rubella or the German measles her mother had contracted when she was pregnant with Linda. Linda had been in and out of the hospital at West Haverstraw over the span of her 18 years, and had undergone a number of corrective operations during that time. Linda and I nearly crossed paths in 1969, a year when we both were at West Haverstraw, but I left the hospital just before Thanksgiving that year whereas Linda arrived just after that. Now here we both were again two years later, and at the same time during this stay. We soon got to know each other and from there our relationship continued to grow.

From the start there was a natural attraction between us. We enjoyed being together and felt at ease with one other. And, we seemed to be perfect supplements to each other's characteristics and needs. Nevertheless, until I made a clear decision about Joyce my relationship with Linda remained uncertain. As in '69, once again I found myself in the midst of two relationships about which to think and make choices, and once again my injury would ultimately and inescapably determine which way I would go.

Ongoing growing ties to and a deepening bond with Joyce depended on the uninterrupted continuation of my pre-injury life, but I didn't have a pre-injury life anymore. Realistically, my accident split my world into two irreconcilable parts—it ended one life, as if wiping a slate clean, and started another that was entirely and unrecognizably different. Although my decision about Joyce had gone right to the verge of going her way, when I looked into the mirror the face of my new identity stared back at me and kept me from carrying it through.

Still, my relationship with Joyce had grown from the bond of friendship we were originally given. True friendship ties are a God-given gift that, despite changes of life circumstance, endure and are not broken. Although the chasm between my pre-injury and post-injury lives could not be bridged, I would continue to value and appreciate this special gift.

In going forward in the new and unknown life before me, I began directing more and more attention toward Linda. Influences from the past would no longer determine the course of my relationship with her. What Linda would be to me she would be on her own merit, given the personal qualities I saw her as having. It was a new time, a time when the unfolding of whatever lay ahead in my *real* post-injury life was to be.

My interest in Linda became more focused. When family members came to West Haverstraw to visit one weekend, a good part of an afternoon away from the hospital was spent hunting for some flowers to take back to Linda. They were carnations and from then on became Linda's favorite flower because of their special meaning to her.

When I went to the Nanuet Mall on one of my regular shopping trips, I ventured into a novelty store and bought Linda a large stuffed mouse that she named "Rasputin." Out of several stuffed mice piled together in a heap, I spotted one with a red, pin-on button saying "I Love You" and knew right away that was the one I wanted to give to Linda.

Linda came up with a more creative and adventurous way of making her feelings about me known. One weekend night as a band was performing in the hospital auditorium, Linda got them to back her in singing the Teddy Bears' "To Know Him is to Love Him" for me. From then on this was "our song," because whenever we heard it after that it had special meaning for us.

Linda was somewhat like Sue had been when Sue came to West Haverstraw back in '69. Linda didn't wait for me to overcome whatever hesitancy and passiveness I might have had, but instead went right ahead and related to me pretty much the way she wanted. She wasn't the type to just sit back and wait for me to maintain the initiative, because I could be lax in that regard. And this was the right approach, since for the most part I went along with how Linda wanted our relationship to be.

Also like Sue, but to a much more limited extent than Sue in her heightened sense of femininity had been, Linda believed in an ordinary romantic relationship that included physical closeness. Sitting on my lap, kissing and embracing were a part of relating to one another while we were together evenings.

139

When the weather was still good, at night we would go outside into the inner court area to have some privacy. As the weather got cooler, we often spent time evenings in the isolated outpatient clinic area of the hospital. The nighttime private refuge of the outpatient clinic area, with all its alcoves and inner corridors and rooms, did not go unnoticed. It became a sanctuary for couples just wanting to be off alone by themselves for a while spending quiet and meaningful time together, and as a "lovers' lane" of sorts saw its share of activity at night.

Not content with where my life was going at home, stirrings within me had brought me back to West Haverstraw for a purpose unknown to me. I could sense something positive before me, yet could not clearly identify it. Preparing to restart my life following my discharge from the hospital, competing opportunities involving not only Joyce and Linda but also hospital staff with whom I had developed interactions made it difficult to determine which path I was meant to follow.

I wasn't sure just what lay ahead in my relationship with Linda, but knew its future course very much depended on Linda herself and how strong her belief was in what she truly wanted for her life. Without complete certainty that Linda had no doubts whatsoever about me being part of the future she was seeking, I would be cautious and hesitant in too actively making set decisions about the outcome of our relationship.

One thing I did know was that after my discharge from the hospital I would be heading to Florida. It would be the end of the year by then and I would be ready for a warm and snow-free climate. I wasn't going to endure any more winters in the North, cooped up inside most of the time.

I had already talked to head nurse Alan, and he seemed enthused by the idea of going to Florida with me. He said the afternoon shift female head nurse from Ward G&H, Chris, might also agree to go with us. The house in Orlando acquired during the summer was vacant and ready for habitation. Orlando had a large medical center to which Alan and Chris could transfer and, with Kennedy Space Center to the east fueling the growth of recently established Florida Technological University, which would later become the University of Central Florida, plus the pending opening of nearby Disney World, Orlando was poised to burgeon as a city of the future.

Alan had a unique way of introducing Chris to me. I was in Ward E&F nurses' station early one warm summer evening talking to Alan. Suddenly Alan commented, "I want you to meet someone," and started heading outside onto the ward's patio. Directly above our ward was Ward G&H, and its nurses' station was directly above that of E&F. At first I wondered where Alan was going and what he was up to. I couldn't figure out what he was doing, but I followed him outside anyway. Then he cleared up the mystery by calling up to the open G&H nurses' station window, "Hey Chris, hang out the window!" With that an attractive young brunette nurse magically appeared at the window and with a broad, pleasant smile leaned out of it to talk with us. Introducing Chris.

I got to know Chris better than just seeing her at the window, because on nights when Alan was off duty she often worked on Ward E&F. I liked having her assist me in getting into bed at night because of the transfer method she used. Usually, when other people helped me into bed I just hooked my arm through a trapeze apparatus and swung myself into bed while someone lifted my feet onto the bed at the same time. Sometimes if I wanted to rest while Linda was on the ward, I would just use a transfer board to shift unto the bed while Linda stood guard in front of me in case I lost my balance. Chris's way was the pivot transfer, and she did it very easily.

Chris could get me to stand straight up and even stay that way for a bit if she wanted. While I was still sitting she would stand in front of me, place my feet close together, and then brace my knees together with her legs. Next she would bend the top part of her body forward and have me put my arms around her shoulders. Then, when she put her arms around my lower back and pulled forward as she straightened up, my leg and lower back muscles would tighten and I would stand right up. With my knees locked and braced by Chris and her arms pressing inward against my lower back, I could remain standing. From that position it was a cinch to pivot and then just sit right down on the bed.

Although I preferred Chris, Alan could do a similar transfer with me. In his smart aleck way, Alan would get me to a standing position and then ask, "May I have this dance?" I think that in choosing a dance partner, I would opt every time for Ginger Rogers rather than Fred Astaire.

Linda had initially been admitted to the hospital to have foot surgery. After surgery she was fitted with a cast, and after physical therapy training was given a pair of crutches and sent home. I soon heard talk among the hospital personnel, though, that Linda was being readmitted to the hospital because she had a hard time using the crutches at home while her foot healed and had fallen. If this was so, it meant I would soon be seeing her again.

Linda did come back to the rehab center, and was given a wheelchair to use until it was time to remove her leg cast. Using the chair in the open halls of the hospital was much easier than trying to get around on crutches in the limited space of her Brooklyn apartment.

If Linda returned home again, one of the options discussed for her for the upcoming year was enrolling at Rockland Community College near West Haverstraw. By now, though, Linda had turned 19 and was ready to move on to a different life she had already chosen. Like me, it was time for her too to set out in her own independent life and she had decided what that was going to be. Linda knew what she wanted for her future and once she put her mind to something she wasn't the type to easily give up on that or be persuaded otherwise.

Although Linda was a determined person in the things she did, this quality didn't outdo her outgoing personality and lively sense of humor. She never let things get too dull, and her wit usually was at the ready whenever it was needed. Linda wasn't one to have to be told to "lighten up." Whenever others lacked enthusiasm, she had enough to go around.

In height Linda was only 4'11", whereas night supervisor Bob was 6'8". Linda liked to kid Bob about being so tall. I was with Linda on her ward one night when Bob started to walk though the doorway of the ward. Linda yelled, "Look out!" and Bob quickly ducked instinctively.

Linda started laughing and a stunned Bob could only reply, "Okay, Linda!" Bob cleared the doorways, but not by much. Still, if there was one person who could make him doubt that, it was Linda.

My stay at West Haverstraw was winding down, and I was discharged from the hospital on Wednesday, December 8, once again under unexpected circumstances. My participation in the drug research study had been completed, so there was no medical reason for me to remain any longer at the hospital. My concern now was finishing my two educational classes, but at grand rounds that morning the social worker pointed out that this would have to take second place to having a medical reason for staying. I said I could leave, but not before the weekend because of having to arrange transportation back to Western New York State. Alan was aware of my upcoming discharge and had offered to drive me home on the weekend, so as far as I was concerned that's the way things stood. He and I needed to finalize plans for the move to Florida.

I went off the ward and took the elevator upstairs to the main part of the hospital so I could phone home with the news about the discharge. The social worker, however, had already called there, saying I had been discharged from the hospital and advising that someone be sent to pick me up. So, at this very moment family members were on their way to West Haverstraw to do just that.

It wasn't the most convenient time to be discharged, because the weekend was just two days away and a weekend discharge would have been much more practical from a transportation standpoint. The trip home was a 400-mile, 8-hour, cross-state drive. A round trip was double that. Whether Alan or family members, a required midweek trip was going to cause someone to have to take time off work. There wasn't much I could do now, though, except go back to the ward and start packing my things.

Earlier at the Physical Therapy Department, in commenting on my upcoming departure from the hospital my therapist Kathy had asked, "What about your friend?" obviously referring to Linda.

I replied, "What about her?"

I really didn't have an answer to Kathy's question. Linda and I had an involvement, but the reality was that I was being discharged from the hospital and that meant our relationship as it had been at West Haverstraw would essentially end when I left. I had for some time now been at a stage in my life where in the right situation with the right person marriage could easily come about. As for Linda, though, I didn't have a set intention to approach her with this in mind because of my need to be sure of the depth and strength of belief of her true feelings.

Very much in the forefront in my mind was the realization that there would be challenges ahead for anyone who married me. After all, I did have a spinal cord injury with accompanying physical limitations. So, in any possible marriage situation I wanted to avoid any uncertainty whatsoever on the other person's part. I wouldn't turn away from marriage if absolute seriousness and certainty about it were made known to me, but without that I would not be actively pursuing or proposing it. If Linda was absolutely sure and determined that our future together was what she wanted and I saw that she had no doubts about it, then even if I left West Haverstaw I would be back for her.

I needn't have wondered about Linda. She was sure about what she wanted and had made up her mind to not let me leave the hospital without asking her to marry me. When I left the ward and was heading for the telephone, I ran into Linda. She stuck around while I phoned home, and then I told her I had been discharged and would be leaving as soon as family members arrived. She said to follow her, and took me to the private room just off Ward A&B that she had been assigned during this last part of her stay at the rehab center. When we were behind closed doors in her room Linda confronted me with, "Well, are you going to ask me?"

This truly was decision time. There wasn't any good reason to not marry her, because to be truthful I was ready to take that step. It was what Linda wanted and she clearly let me know that. There weren't any hesitations or doubts on her part, and I saw that as an indication that she was serious about it. It seemed like getting married was something we were both about as ready as ever to do if we were going to do it. There wasn't much else to do at this point than go ahead with it. Tentatively I asked, "Do you want to?" but I already knew the answer.

Whatever my physical limitations now were, there were no boundaries to my ability to commit to a lasting relationship. I could determine the quality of my commitment, and this very important choice was something I did have to offer. No matter how much I had messed up in the past, marriage was one thing I had a chance to do the right way. I still had control of the rest of my life, and it was time to start living it more wisely and correctly. Marriage would be a new start. I was ready for it and it was the right thing to do. Other than being restored to full physical health once again, getting married probably was the best thing that could have happened to me at this point in my life.

Linda wanted a marriage commitment, and that's what she got. We came out of her room as two people promised to each other, and 10 days later I returned to West Haverstraw and was married to her in the hospital auditorium by the hospital's Protestant chaplain. My brother-in-law Gary stood as best man, and Linda's father was there to give her away. Linda may have had doubts when first I dropped her wedding ring and then ran over her bridal train, but she didn't change her mind.

The ceremony was quite an event, to which a packed auditorium of patients, staff, relatives and even the press, attested. Of special meaning was the beautiful wedding cake the hospital kitchen staff had labored hard to prepare as a wedding gift. It was large and layered, but because of its height it was leaning a bit to one side. It didn't fall, though, and they did a great job for not being professional cake makers. Besides, it was a gift from the heart.

After the wedding, as a married couple now Linda and I set out traveling with family members back to Royalton Center in Western New York State to spend the Christmas holidays before leaving to set up our own home in Florida. We stopped overnight in Binghamton, because the entire trip couldn't be made that evening. The first floor of the hotel we stayed at was all booked, so everyone took rooms on the second floor. This made accessibility a bit more difficult since there wasn't an elevator available to us, but we managed. There were enough people in our group that it wasn't too much of a problem. We found a fine Italian restaurant nearby and had good food, drink and more celebration.

Our marriage presented a unique opportunity that would make possible a successful and rewarding life for both Linda and myself. Each of us was in a situation where alone the future was questionable but because of the complementing qualities we shared, together we had a chance to make something of our lives. We supplemented well each other's needs and limitations, and united were two people possessing a lot of potential.

By joining together we could achieve the freedom and independence we needed. Our strength was in teaming together, because our combining assets enabled us to reach for goals that might not have otherwise been obtainable. Working together, there probably wasn't too much that was going to stop us from getting out of life what we could. If ever the whole was stronger than its two separate parts, this was it.

One very important thing I didn't have to worry about in our relationship was Linda's reaction to my physical limitations, because all of her life many of her closest relations had been with persons having one type of physical condition or another, and also she herself was no stranger to physical problems. So, what might have been a factor with someone else wasn't a factor at all with Linda.

Marrying Linda was the right thing to do. Although I had concern about ever again finding someone as devoted as Joyce, very fortunately Linda had a similar dedication. She told me her purpose and aim was to help me achieve whatever goals I had in life, and that her support would always be there. It wasn't one-sided, though. My presence and support were also important in allowing Linda to realize her full potential and to get from life a lot of things she wasn't sure she would get the chance to experience or obtain.

While in my pre-injury life it was unlikely that anyone could have matched Joyce's personality and natural suitability, it would have been hard for anyone to top Linda in my post-injury life. A guy is lucky if he finds one truly dedicated woman during his lifetime. I came across two, but maybe that's because my life was cut into two separate parts at the time of my accident so I had one more coming. The accident definitely was about as down on my luck as I could have gotten at that point in my life. Nonetheless, from there making the most of what was still left was due largely to the presence of Linda.

Despite any differences Linda and I might have had as separate individuals, and our internal characteristics were very different, we functioned well as a team. We respected each other and took one another's interests in mind. We didn't believe in destructive negative influences such as unnecessary conflict in marriage, so we agreed early that anything beyond positive give-and-take expressions of our individual views would not be part of our relationship. This wasn't hard to do, because what we both had already experienced in our lives had taught us the difference between things of real importance and those about which to not be too concerned.

Besides this, though, a relationship of shared dependency brings with it a realization of just how indispensable the other person is and makes each partner truly appreciate the value of the other. Recognizing the value of a relationship is something important that sees no relevance in the unnecessary influence of negative things that could diminish the quality and meaning of the union. There are more important aspects of life on which to focus than trivial differences that really should be kept in proper perspective.

Marriage begins with a mutually felt love, but requires much more to keep growing and thriving. That additional key to a positive marriage for Linda and myself was a genuine dedication to the quality and success of our relationship, along with mutual acceptance, respect and unconditional support. And, of course, total self-interest won't work in any relationship so a certain amount of sacrifice and giving priority to one another's needs also was important.

Linda was the partner I needed. With her I could regain some of the control over my life I had lost. She would become an important part of my new self-identity, and over the course of time our reliance on each another would result in the two of us becoming even more united. This was mainly a positive thing. The only negative aspect was the consequences it would have for either of us if anything ever happened to the other.

XVIII. Starting Over

January 10, 1972 marked the beginning of a new life. Linda and I left snowy Western New York State and arrived in the warm 80-degree sunshine of Central Florida. Here we would make our new home. Here we would begin our journey forward. And, here we would have the start we needed.

Nestled at the end of a short sandy lane, the continuation of which was stopped by a thick stand of woods, our location on the eastern outskirts of Orlando was quiet and countryish yet close to the more urban area to the west.

We needed transportation to get to places, so a priority was the purchase of a car. We found a cute, little new '72 Chevy Camaro glittering with an eye-catching finish of brown metallic paint, and its size suited Linda perfectly. After a few driving lessons, she passed her driver's test and had a license. Yet we Northerners soon found that a car without air-conditioning wasn't the best choice when living in Florida, and also transfers in and out of it weren't the easiest for me.

By fall we switched to a new, full-size '73 Buick Centurion with air-conditioning and 6-way power seats that provided both comfort and ease of transfers. We had the Buick modified and I began driving too, but this and my past driving record didn't impress Linda and she preferred to be the one behind the wheel.

Eventually we would find that a van with an automatic lift was the most practical means of transportation. It eliminated repeated wheelchair transfers required when using a car.

With our new opportunity before us, I thought I had left much of the conflict of my pre-injury/post-injury life behind. Distance alone, though, does not guarantee such a haven. Bad news from the North came, and suddenly it all cascaded right down on me again. March 17, 1972—the day of my 26th birthday and last day of my brother Ray's life. In his fierce internal struggle to make sense of the extreme contradictions of his recent life experiences, Ray reached the point where mentally he was too overwhelmed to cope with the emotional pain of living anymore. The news of his death was yet another reminder that life, for all it has to offer, can still be a harsh place where anything can happen. It had happened to me, and now in a much worse and final way it had happened to Ray. Was ours the inevitable "don't be so sure" fate of two young guys who once thought the world was their playground and a place where they were in complete control?

Our similarities in my pre-injury years were similarities of a different sort now. Life had showed us how wrong we were. We lived life our way, but at a cost too high to pay. Our brief storming of life was an excessive high that burned out like a crashing meteor. We thought we had control, but we never did. We were on the wrong course and didn't see it. And when you don't see where you're going, you fall off the precipice. We were doomed, because we couldn't admit there was a better way than ours.

The timing of Ray's death bothered me. There was too much symbolism. Being older, I was a role model for Ray and someone he wanted to be like. To him my injury was like a bubble bursting, and symbolically it was the death of the approach to life I had so strongly embraced, because now look what was left of all those illusions. It invalidated the vision of life Ray had seen through me. The accident happened when I was 22, about 10 weeks short of my 23rd birthday. Now Ray was gone at age 22, about 10 weeks short of his 23rd birthday, and right at a time that for him represented not a celebration of life for me but rather all that had been lost.

Other factors, building one on top of another, added their weight, including horrendous experiences as a combat Marine in Vietnam. In a very short period of time, Ray's idealism did a complete turnaround. Unkind things began to occur that weren't supposed to in the world he used to believe in. In Ray's world young people didn't get injured or die, yet in an uninterrupted series of events that's what happened.

Still, the effect of the relationship between Ray and me was not to be underestimated. It was the master brick in the foundation of our view of the world around us. We shared a unique approach to life that, while unrealistic and short-lived, bound us together in an inseparable way. Something couldn't happen to me without affecting Ray, because his identity and outlook were so closely linked to mine that there had to be some internal consequence.

Ray was disillusioned when he realized our idyllic image of life had been a mirage. After the accident, we each had serious consequences with which to deal—Ray psychologically and me both physically and psychologically. I kept plodding along, even though it was tough facing my dramatically changed life, and Ray kept plodding until he couldn't plod any longer.

The total change after the accident we had was the starting point of the downward spiral Ray continued to experience. There were reasons why Ray felt guilt following that night, which we never talked through, just as there were in his mind reasons for the guilt he felt when he was confronted by the subsequent deaths of others— ranging from very close and important to not acquaintances at all. Guilt, when not knowing how to deal with it, can be a very self-destructive inner force.

Inner feelings are strange and powerful forces that are not rational or easily controlled. They are what overpowered Ray, but we can all look at ourselves at times and see these kinds of forces at work within us, with some being more powerful and uncontrollable than others.

The loss of Ray was a loss of another part of myself, since we had so closely identified with each other and had been so similar in so many ways. Ray was now gone, along with the worldly burdens he had such a hard time carrying. Over time there would be other tragic losses of family members to face, but none would have for me the same inescapable dynamics as did Ray's loss.

Yet regardless of all that had happened and how devastating it was, it was now time to put everything behind and look ahead with the new hope and optimism I had originally brought with me to Florida. I had another chance at life, and it was up to me to try to rise above previous trials and tragedies, because as much as I wanted I couldn't go back and change anything for me, Ray, or anyone else. I had to go forward with my focus on the future. Once more I had control to make the right decisions and influence my destiny to the extent to which I set my mind.

It couldn't be denied that by making wrong choices earlier my life had been irretrievably transformed. The boundless euphoria of two previously undefeatable guys had forever vanished and was no more to be found in this world. But it was now a new and different time, one much more realistic, and even though so much had changed that it was hard accepting that me and Ray once had all we did and then lost it, my present responsibility was building a positive and fulfilling life with Linda and achieving all we could.

Since graduating from high school in the summer of '64, I had attended four colleges and still not completed my bachelor's degree. The summer of '72 provided Linda and me some much-needed getaway time with family and friends in Western New York State. Upon returning to Florida in the fall, I enrolled at the University of Central Florida on the rural eastern outskirts of Orlando and there finally completed my bachelor of arts degree in psychology as well as two years of graduate study in clinical psychology. Then it was on to Tampa where I began study in the rehabilitation counseling master's degree program at the University of South Florida. I soon switched to the graduate program in sociology after being offered a research assistant position in that department, and stayed on until completing my master of arts degree in sociology.

Having started off in Orlando and then moving to Tampa, Linda and I next set our sights on Gainesville where the University of Florida was located. I was accepted into the doctorate degree program in sociology there, and worked for the sociology department as a teaching and research assistant. In addition to getting my Ph.D. degree in medical sociology, I also earned a graduate certificate in gerontology, the study of aging, from UF's Center for Gerontological Studies while working there as a research assistant. I found time to do tutoring for the University Athletic Association, working with UF's men and women athletes. I enjoyed the more personal interaction that one-on-one and small-group teaching provided.

Linda also became involved with the university, working at the Center for Gerontological Studies, the Department of Psychology, and the School of Medicine's Department of Pediatrics.

Having limitations that had changed my physical interaction with the world around me, I had set mental goals and reached them by going as high in my level of education as I could. My next goals were to advance my personal and spiritual development to reflect what I felt was the primary purpose for my existence in and journey through this world.

Of course, the progress of spinal cord injury research and treatment also was a primary issue for me. I became an area consultant and counselor in the social, psychological and environmental aspects for a number of national groups. When a chance came to participate in a research study at the Miami Project to Cure Paralysis, Linda and I temporarily moved to Miami. Being in Miami gave us an opportunity to see just how far spinal cord injury research was progressing.

Encouraged by the amount of funding and effort being applied to spinal cord regeneration research, we returned to Gainesville where the University of Florida's spinal cord regeneration program became one of the priorities at the newly established Brain Institute. In Miami, Gainesville and elsewhere both nationally and internationally, accomplishments in spinal cord injury regeneration research were becoming more and more promising. Enhanced soft tissue imaging, molecular biology, and genetic engineering were bringing researchers ever closer to reversing the devastating physical effects of spinal cord injury.

153

RONALD C. SCHULTZ, PH.D.

So, here me and Linda were. Transplanted from the harsher climate of New York State we became homeowners in the sunny South, eventually settling in Ocala in the midst of the scenic thoroughbred horse county of North Central Florida—two people with uncertain futures who met in a rehabilitation center, got married there, and then set out to see if we could build a successful and rewarding life together in the outside world. Through determination and teamwork we succeeded, and learned much about life along the way.

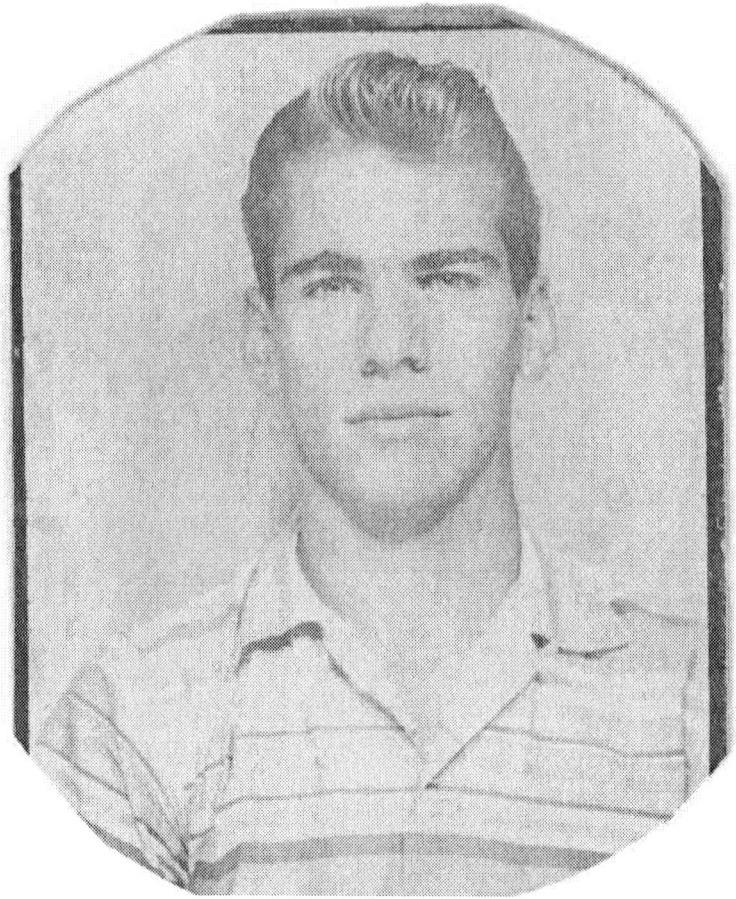

Ron, 1967/68

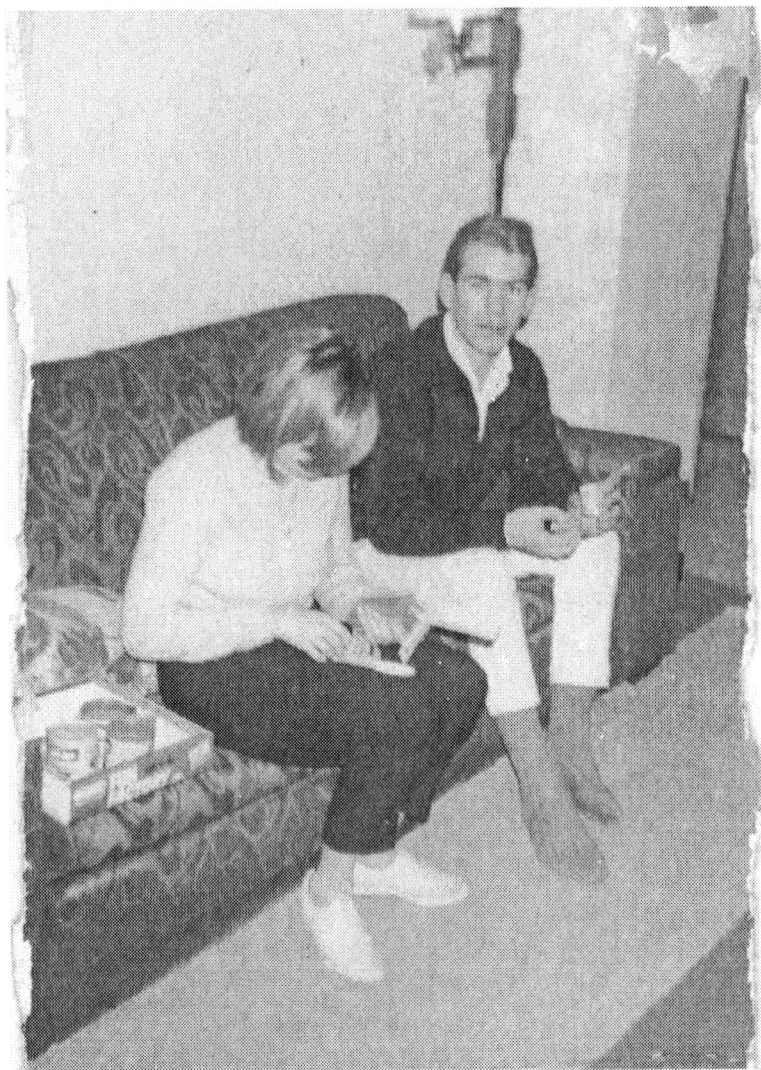

Ron and Joyce, early 1967

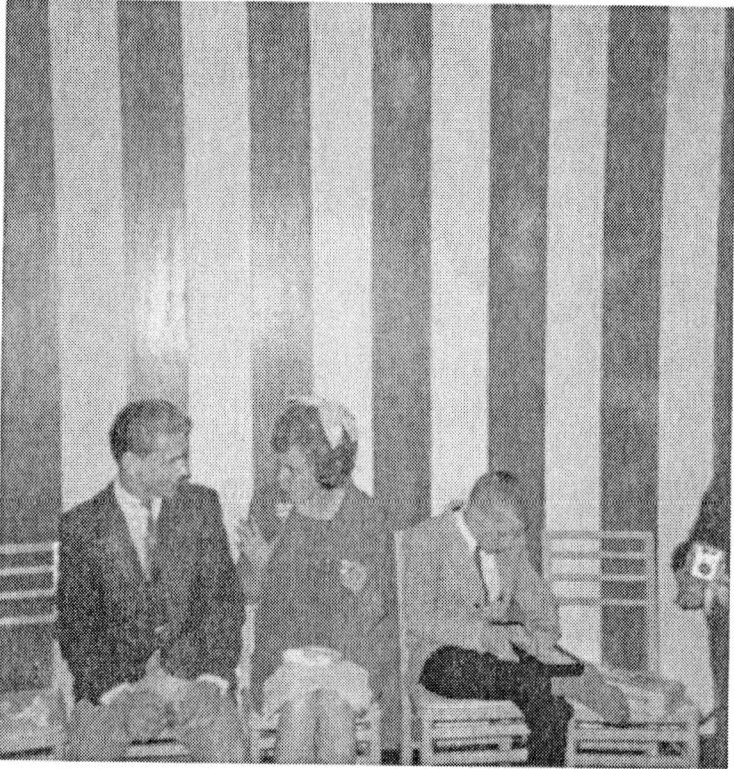

Ron, aunt and cousin at relative's wedding reception, Springfield, Illinois, June 1967

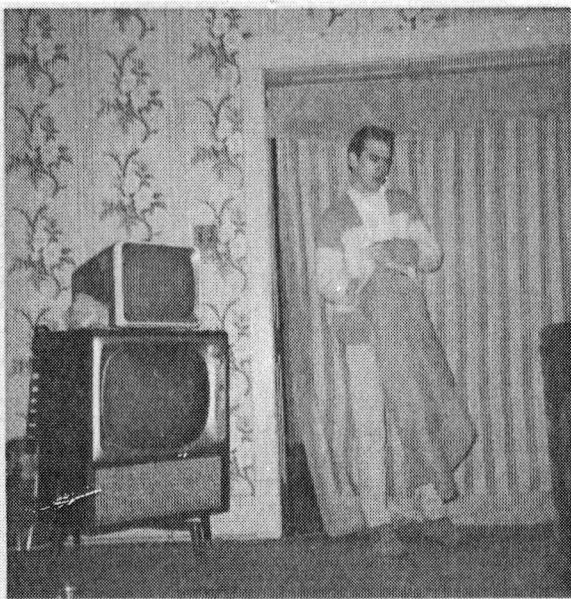

Ron while student at Valparaiso University, Valparaiso, Indiana, March 1968

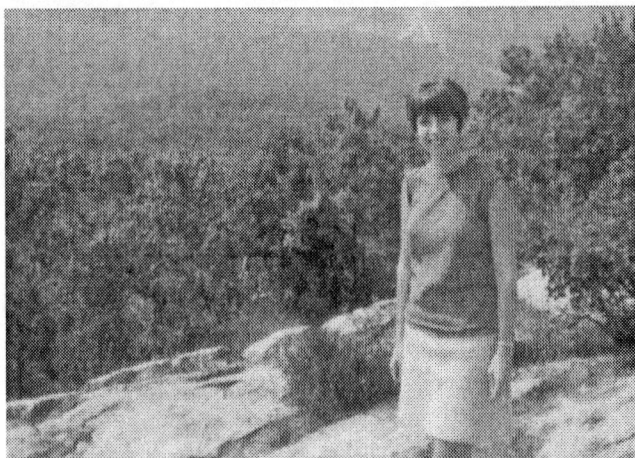

Joyce, West Haverstraw, fall 1969

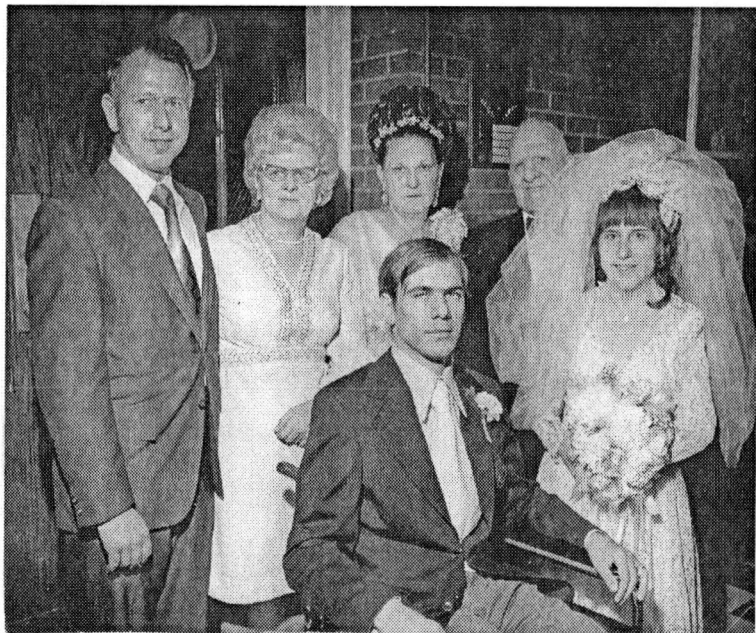

Wedding, Ron and Linda with parents, December 1971

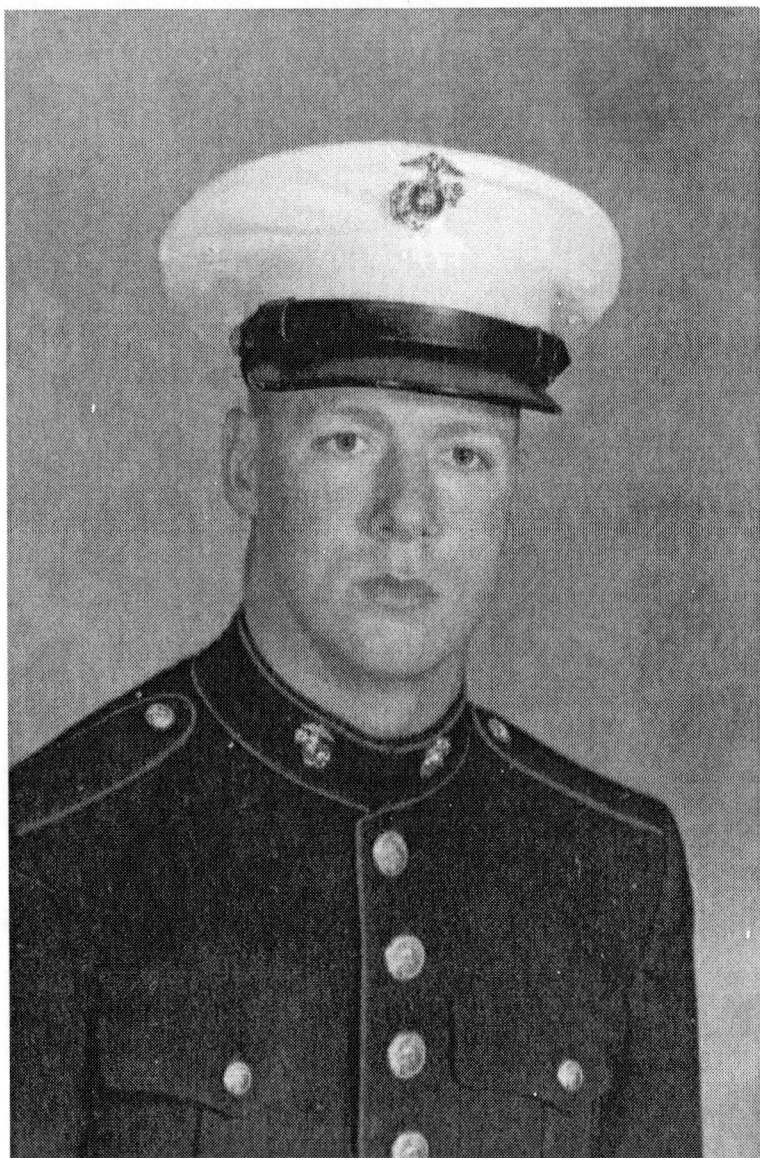

Brother Ray in Marine dress, 1970

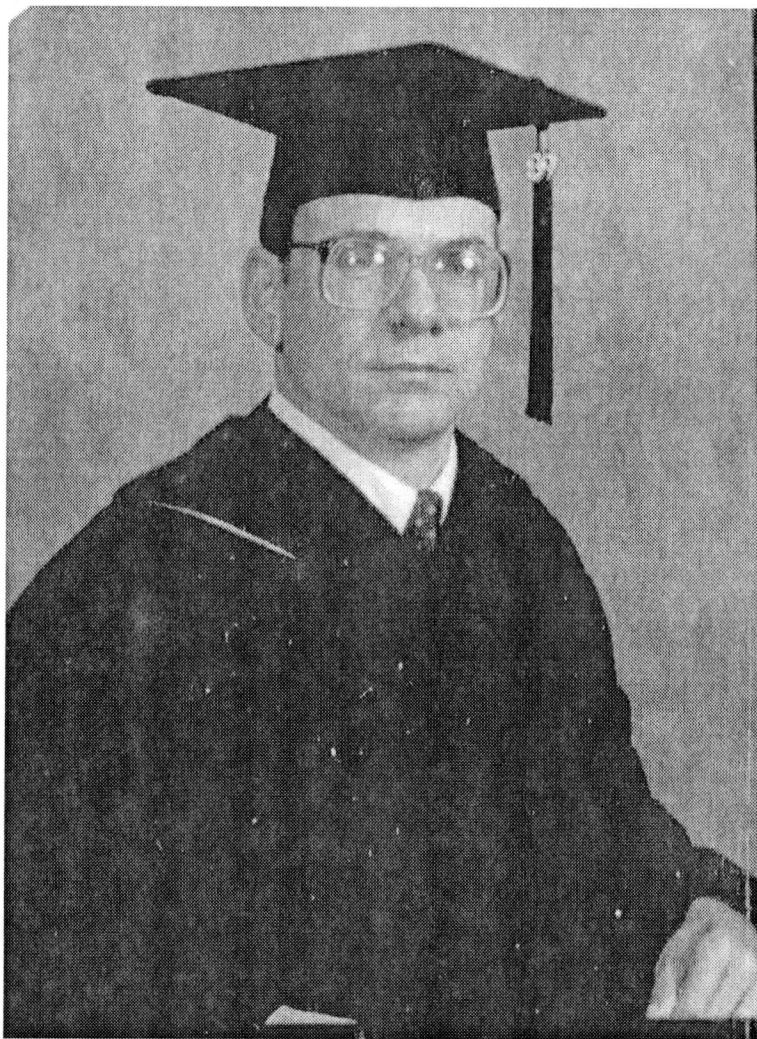

Ron, doctorate degree graduation, University of Florida, Gainesville, 1989

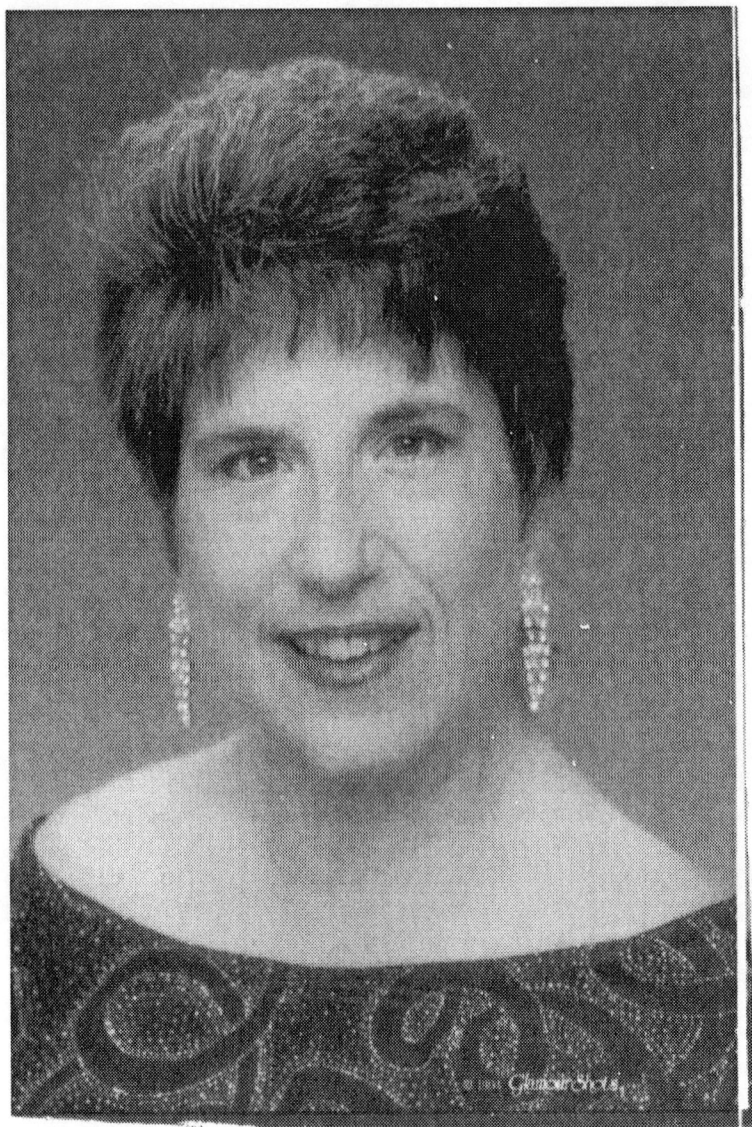

Linda, Gainesville, Florida, early 1990s

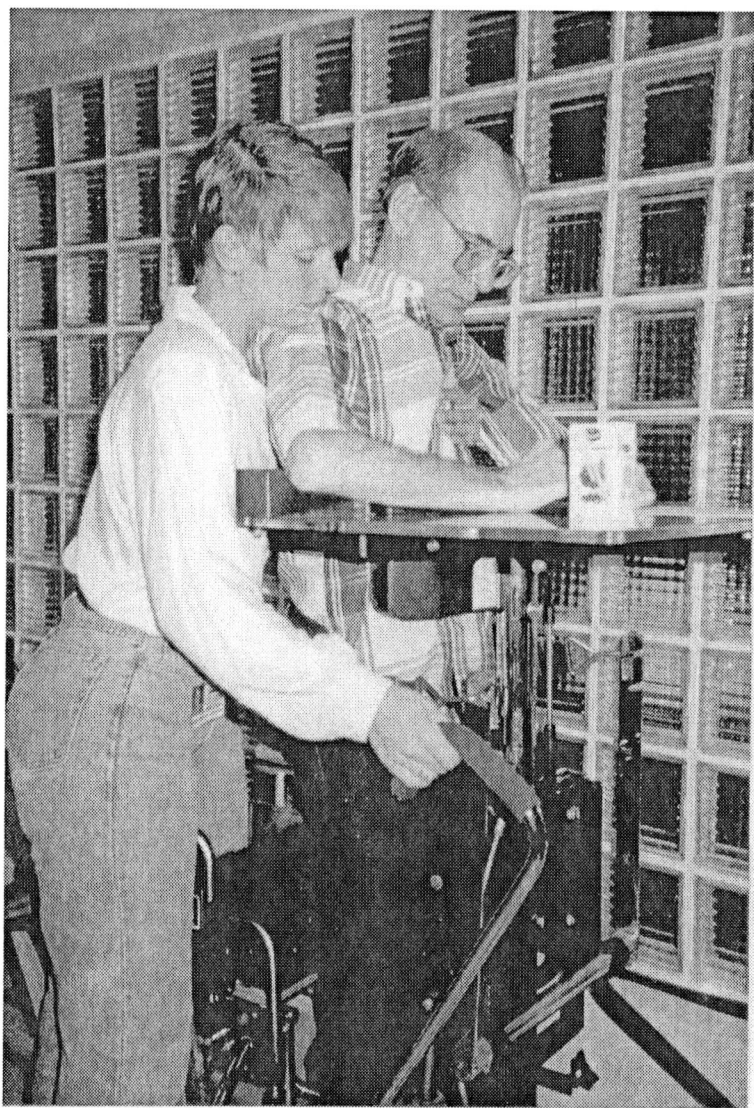

Ron while at Miami Project participating in research study, Miami, Florida, 1992

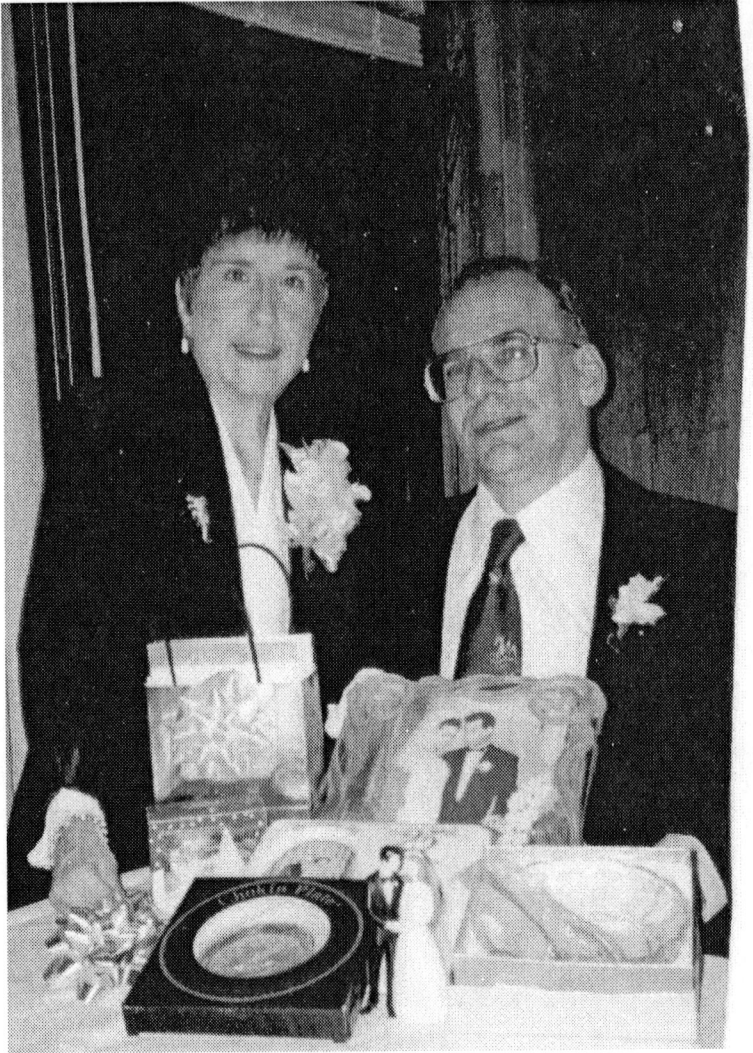

Ron and Linda, 25th wedding anniversary, December 1996

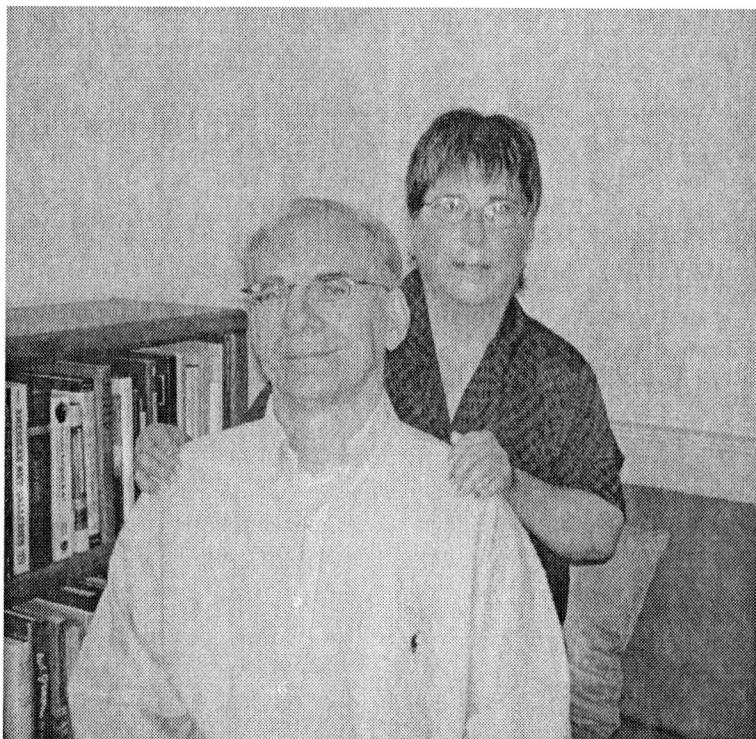

Ron and Linda, Ocala, Florida, December 2005

XIX. A Final Word

To every thing there is a season,
and a time to every purpose under heaven.

Holy Bible, Ecclesiastes 3:1

This was a difficult chapter to write, and you surely would not be reading this story had my life taken a different turn. Life, though, does not always go the way we want or expect. Along the way there are trials and challenges, some being more serious and life-changing than others. So here I am, telling about a single, momentary event that altered the entire course of my existence. Suddenly and unexpectedly, I was left to wonder. What had happened to the limitless potential of youth that before had been right there in front of me? Had everything ended? Could I salvage anything and have any kind of rewarding and fulfilling life at all?

At first, answers didn't come easily. It was hard getting past the feeling that life had passed me by—that I had missed out on so many things that were yet ahead of me before my accident. My injury took away so much physical capability that I could experience only a small part of what I had the potential to experience before it. I felt I couldn't live life to the fullest with the physical limitations I had.

There would be a rough road ahead. We do live in a physical world and physical capability is important, not only to help make everyday living easier but also because psychologically and socially physical health is important for our own self-image and the image others have of us. When spinal cord injury occurs at an early age, as it usually does, it makes things even harder because so much of life that still lies ahead has to be faced with a tremendous physical, psychological and social disadvantage.

It was a struggle to not dwell on the downside of life that follows spinal cord injury, and tough to stay focused on the positive things that still could be had afterward. It is unrealistic to pretend that spinal cord injury does not drastically alter the future course of one's life, but it also is self-defeating to get stuck too negatively on an event that cannot be taken back and must be made the best of by moving forward and getting the most out of what yet remains.

Because realistically I had to, I did *adjust* to my injury in my everyday living the best I could so I would have some quality of post-injury life. Yet, it was something that inwardly I never fully *accepted*. Although outwardly I didn't give up and stop living, not one day went by when I wished my accident had never happened. Inside I just couldn't accept the self-identity of a spinal cord injured person. My spirit was too free and wouldn't allow that. It wasn't going to change, though, so I had to make the best of it. It would take time, faith, hope, belief, determination and the support of others to help me realize that with the right thinking and actions the most important goals in life could still be reached.

When my life in this world began it started with God-given gifts I should have cherished, respected and safeguarded. But as time went by, through freedom of choice I made life decisions that were not the right ones and that led to a lifestyle that eventually could have only negative consequences. The negative consequences did come, but I was spared mortal injury and given a second chance. God looked into my heart and saw the potential to get it right and find the life purpose intended for me. I was given more gifts, only now things would not be as easy with the physical restrictions of my post-injury life.

So, how can the challenges of living with spinal cord injury or similar conditions be overcome? Part of the answer lies in the strength and determination within us. Support of family and others is important too. Yet, above all else is faith in the Higher Being that each person chooses or not to embrace. I am a Christian, and my belief has been a strong, sustaining force that has kept me focused and forward-guided and has been the ultimate source of my life's purpose and meaning.

The reason family and others are a key factor is we are social beings who in our daily living are not isolated from the world around us. Clearly, there is more than one victim when spinal cord injury occurs. Suddenly and unexpectedly the lives of those close to anyone facing a spinal cord injury are affected to a large extent too.

First, there are immediate concerns. Right after my accident family and others feared I might not even survive. When that threat passed they were then faced with the uncertainty of just how much recovery I would have. Entire relationship patterns changed as my post-injury life, a completely new and different life, began to unfold. Inescapably, the lives of others were very much impacted simply because of my ties to them.

Spinal cord injury can happen to anyone at any time. Most unfortunate are those it happens to through no direct fault of their own. In other cases, risky or irresponsible behavior may be the cause. We come into this world with a special gift—freedom of choice. This is what helps define us as human beings and gives us the opportunity to get the most out of life. Yet, with this gift comes the responsibility to use our choices wisely and in the right way. The outcomes we encounter as we go through life are largely the result of the decisions we make and the way we live.

We have to be careful with our life choices, because once a major mistake is made it may not be possible to undo. Often, there is little room for error. It is wise to heed the warning, "A prudent person foresees the danger ahead and takes precautions; the simpleton goes blindly on and suffers the consequences." (Holy Bible, Proverbs 22:3)

To have meaning and inspiration for others, I realized the final message of my story had to be about the purposeful and good things that come from life—things such as the lessons and growth we are put here to have during our life's journey. Regardless of what happens along the way and what we must endure, our task is to prove ourselves and become worthy of a life beyond that will be much more lasting and fulfilling.

The biblical verse at the beginning of this chapter sums up the course of our life experiences in this physical world. There is indeed a set time for each experience during life's journey. What changes this given pattern for all, though, are the actions we take along the way because of our freedom of choice and also life occurrences that come along regardless of what actions we consciously take. My story is one of life choices, while the experiences of others faced with serious life challenges may be ones of life misfortune that came regardless of choices made.

Everyone has his or her own particular burdens to bear, depending on their degree and nature. We are clearly told that is how life in this world will be—"In the world ye shall have tribulation" (Holy Bible, John 16:33)—and it is up to us to meet, endure and rise above those challenges. If we do that, then we win in the end and gain what is meant for us. That is the intended life course set before us. No matter what freedom we think we may have in this world, an even greater freedom lies beyond. Everyday life shows that the physical world is not permanent, which means something else is. Cultivating that "something else" within will reap its own final reward.

In the meantime the physical world, despite its impermanence and uncertainties, marches on and medical science marches on. As they look ahead in their lives, this gives hope to those seeking refuge from the binding chains of spinal cord injury and similar afflictions that are so limiting.

At the time of my accident, medicine could do little to reverse or improve spinal cord injury. Spinal cord injured persons have not had other alternatives besides just living with their condition. But it is now a new millennium, and things are changing.

In time a cure for spinal cord injury will come. Much more effective medical treatment immediately following injury is already here. With the technology that continues to develop, a cure for spinal cord injury cure is no longer a question of if but when. Although personal growth as we go through life is a rewarding goal and accomplishment in itself, how much more satisfying it would be to have the added bonus of a well-functioning physical body while pursuing it.

Still, no matter what happens to us physically as we run the gamut from birth to death, there is inside of us a mind, heart, spirit and soul that once developed the way we want cannot be lost. This is where life's true journey is won. We are not here to stagnate or go backward, but to grow and develop to the fullest that inner core that really makes us who we are. Over time we cannot escape physical change and decline, yet the height we reach in our nonphysical quest will endure for all time.

Beyond all that seems negative in spinal cord injury and life in general—physically, psychologically and socially—is a positive and powerful force shining brightly ahead showing the way. Having hope, faith and belief despite all we encounter and keeping our sight on the ultimate goal that is meant for us is what truly matters in the end.

This has been my story, a story of what I experienced and learned. It is a saga of gifts, opportunities, losses, trials and challenges, hope and triumph. Only by stumbling and falling in life can a genuine appreciation and understanding of its true value and meaning be gained. Always look upward, and a guiding light will be there.

Have a good life. It will be what you make of it, and helped by gifts received from above.

RCS

Printed in the United States
68983LVS00007B/29

9 781424 126484